your appetite, body composition, and overall fitness level. The intelligence of *Stress Less, Weigh Less* is its focus on the root problem in our society, chronic stress. It gives us powerful yet practical tools to get our stress under control, leading us back to a healthy body, mind, and spirit."

—DR. KAREN WOLFE, former medical director of Australian Government Health Services, physician, international speaker, author, coach, and leading pioneer in wellness and mind/body health

"Holly has solved the mystery of healthy, permanent weight loss. In her book, *Stress Less, Weigh Less,* she shows us how to use the power of the mind to ensure sustainable weight loss by managing stressful situations that are continually bombarding us. She is a true leader in the health industry and an asset to families everywhere. *Stress Less, Weigh Less* is a must-have book, not just to read, but to live by. I highly recommend it."

—HEATHER W. BRIEN, MD, board-certified general surgeon and board-certified vascular surgeon, American Board of Surgery

"Providing the best guidance I have ever seen, Holly Mosier's book, *Stress Less, Weigh Less,* is a user-friendly manual for a life of health, wellness, and vitality. Holly's book follows the guidance of the Food and Drug Administration, but in a way that is relatable to the average person. While not new wisdom, Holly is able to walk each of us from the point of understanding to intervention and participation on our own behalf. She shows us exactly how to master our fate and add years to our lives. But not just years; quality of life is just as important as duration, if not more. Her book provides the methods for achieving and maintaining health, yet in a reasonable way that can and should be embraced by everyone. I believe Holly's book should be a mandatory read for all of us."

—ALAN O. MARCUS, MD, FACP, FACE, retired associate clinical professor, USC Keck School of Medicine, Division of Endocrinology and Metabolism; director, South Orange County Endocrinology Research Department; and former global director of medical affairs, Medtronic Diabetes

STRESS LESS, WEIGH LESS

FOLLOW HOLLY *to* INCREASE ENERGY,
EAT *the* FOOD YOU LOVE, *and*
ENJOY *an* AGELESS BODY

HOLLY MOSIER

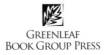

GREENLEAF
BOOK GROUP PRESS

This book is intended as a reference volume only, not as a medical manual. The information given here is designed to help you make informed decisions about your health. It is not intended as a substitute for any treatment that may have been prescribed by your doctor. If you suspect that you have a medical problem, you should seek competent medical help. You should not begin a new health regimen without first consulting a medical professional.

Published by Greenleaf Book Group Press
Austin, Texas
www.gbgpress.com

Distributed by Greenleaf Book Group LLC

For ordering information or special discounts for bulk purchases, please contact Greenleaf Book Group LLC at PO Box 91869, Austin, TX 78709, 512.891.6100.

Design and composition by Greenleaf Book Group LLC and Bumpy Design
Cover design by Greenleaf Book Group LLC
Yoga photos and cover photo: Starla Fortunato
Workout photos: Keith J. Williams
Food and lifestyle photos: Rob Mosier
Beach yoga photo: Moore & Cruz Photography

Publisher's Cataloging-In-Publication Data
(Prepared by The Donohue Group, Inc.)
Mosier, Holly.
  Stress less, weigh less : follow Holly to increase energy, eat the food you love, and enjoy an ageless body / Holly Mosier. — 1st ed.
     p. : ill. ; cm.
  ISBN: 978-1-60832-113-1

  1. Stress—Health aspects. 2. Stress management. 3. Health—Psychological aspects. 4. Weight loss—Psychological aspects. 5. Mind and body. I. Title.

RA785 .M67 2011
613.7   2011923948

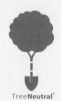

Part of the Tree Neutral® program, which offsets the number of trees consumed in the production and printing of this book by taking proactive steps, such as planting trees in direct proportion to the number of trees used: www.treeneutral.com

Printed in the United States of America on acid-free paper

11 12 13 14 15 16 10 9 8 7 6 5 4 3 2 1

First Edition

CONTENTS

PREFACE

Writing this book has been so much fun, and I am delighted to get it into your hands. It really is my private manual and includes all of my stress-reduction and practical spirituality tools, and eating and exercising guidelines (which are easier, quicker, and more economical than you might think) that have served me very well into middle age . . . and will serve me, I am quite sure, well beyond. Let me tell you how it came about.

There is nothing special about me. I live a very typical Western lifestyle. There is, however, one thing that has made my life special. Several years ago, I decided to change my perspective. Instead of focusing on my limitations, I began to direct my thought to something more exciting and expansive—just to see how it would feel. I began to play a fun mental game of "Wouldn't it be nice if . . . ?" And I filled in those blanks with uplifting and fanciful dreams.

This felt good, so I did more of it.

As I played this mental game again and again, slowly but unmistakably my way of thinking began to change. And as I changed mentally, the external, visible part of me also began to change. The potency of the mind-body connection revealed itself. Not only did I lose weight and gain muscle, I became peaceful. I projected an aura of energy and happiness. I changed so much that people noticed and began to ask me how they could improve their own appearance and find a measure of inner peace without sacrificing the things they loved. They wanted to know how they could look better, feel better, and perform better at whatever they chose to do. I understood that beneath their desire for physical health lay a desire for mental and spiritual health as well. Many of them longed to release themselves from the negative habits of thought that were affecting their bodies, constricting them in their clothes, and making them feel encased and trapped, a daily reminder that they unconsciously accepted limitation instead of insisting on the freedom that would allow them to really thrive.

When I saw the positive impact that I had on people's lives, I decided that I wanted to share what I have learned with as many people as possible. So I decided to write this book. It's my hope that the lessons I have learned can help you transform your body and your mind. You've taken the first step toward a new, invigorated life. The rest is easy. Just follow me.

I KNOW WHY WE'RE GETTING FATTER

We're a nation of fatties—obesity is rising at an alarming rate. In the late 1970s, the Centers for Disease Control and Prevention (CDC) estimated that 47 percent of U.S. adults were either overweight or obese. In 2003–2004, that number rose to 66 percent.[1] By 2009, the CDC called our climbing obesity rate a "national crisis."[2]

Why is this happening? Myriad studies have produced a variety of conclusions. Some say it's our inclusion of food at every event, at every occasion, and on every corner. Some say it results from an increase in our intake of refined carbohydrates and trans fats. Some say that it's a simple matter of ballooning portion sizes.

Other studies have focused on how modern conveniences, such as the TV remote

---

1   CDC, National Center for Health Statistics, "Prevalence of overweight, obesity and extreme obesity among adults: United States, trends 1976–80 through 2005–2006," December 2008.
2   Department of Health and Human Services, CDC, Justification of Estimates for Appropriation Committees, Fiscal Year 2009, p. 13.

control and several cars per family, have allowed us to move less. We don't think twice about driving one block to the grocery store, even if we're just picking up a few things that would be easy to carry on a walk home.

And then there are computers, the Internet, and our smart phones. I don't know about you, but I no longer even get up to check the phone book to find a number; I don't move from the computer—I just type in a search, and the number appears. The kids spend hours on the computer doing homework and playing games rather than going outdoors for a game of kick the can with the neighbor kids, as we used to do in the '60s and '70s. Many people don't even need to move to a computer. They can get the information they need, and all the entertainment they want, on their smart phones wherever they happen to be sitting.

But all those modern conveniences have come with a price: increased stress.

We are literally plugged in 24/7. Gone are the days when we could go home after work, turn it all off, and unwind. Remember those days? No call waiting, no computers, no cell phones, no BlackBerries. The last twenty years have changed all that. Today, we cannot escape the flashing red light of the smart phone commanding us to check the latest e-mail, text, or instant message. Our computers make it too easy to continue work at home after a full day at the office. Then there is social media— Facebook, Twitter—calling to be looked at and responded to. We have become a wired, stressed-out culture. According to innumerable recent studies, our stress levels have increased at an alarming rate, causing numerous health and psychological issues. According to the CDC, *two-thirds* of family doctor visits are now due to stress.

Beyond causing illness, as if that weren't bad enough, all that stress affects our midsections. It causes our endocrine systems to dump excess stress hormones into our bodies—which really does increase our food cravings. It's not your imagination. And with the ease of drive-throughs and instant food, it takes but a moment to soothe any craving with a burger, fries, and a shake.

To me, the reason for our obesity problem is obvious. We move less and eat more. Is it really any mystery? Add to that our ever-increasing stress coupled with the hormonal changes that come in midlife—for men and women both—that genuinely do cause cravings and lethargy, and it makes sense that most of us are chubby, certainly after passing forty.

If we all want to lose weight, and the cause of our weight problem is so obvious, then why is it so hard for people to eat less and move more? I decided that I would find out the answer for myself. And, after years of experimentation, I succeeded. Armed with this knowledge, I declared war on weight gain. And I won.

MY DECADES OF STRUGGLE WITH **WEIGHT CONTROL**

I didn't set out to become a fitness expert or to develop any sort of weight-loss plan. I simply was seeking a holistic solution to that nagging problem of weight control—a solution that would fit into my life in a realistic way without requiring me to relinquish the foods I loved and add more stress to my already hectic life. I didn't know that applying my lifelong study of spiritual principles to my body would transform my body in ways beyond imagination, but that's what ended up happening. It took years, but my passion (okay, obsession) to find this simple solution carried me through. It was a work of joy, a lot of laughter, and many, many frustrating moments as I tested theories and tools on my own body, meticulously recording my results and finally landing on a straightforward, no-nonsense formula that brought my middle-aged body to, by far, the best shape of my life and bestowed a peace of mind that I had never experienced before.

During my late teens to early thirties, I was a working actress. I appeared in soap operas (*Days of Our Lives* and *General Hospital*) and filmed many national commercials, including spots for McDonald's, Canada Dry ginger ale, Chevrolet, Kentucky Fried Chicken, Domino's Pizza, and a Pepsi ad with a then-unknown Heather Locklear. Because of this, I had to meticulously maintain a consistent weight, or the sad fact was I wouldn't get hired. So I kept my weight under control by following a strict pattern of long daily gym workouts and testing every diet that came down the pike, with occasional binges followed by excessive exercising and fasting. Still, I thought my daily diet was basically healthy.

I kicked off most mornings with a homemade raisin oat-bran muffin or a whole-wheat bagel with light cream cheese. Lunch was usually fruit with yogurt or salad. I always ate a big salad at dinner, along with a large baked potato, pasta, veggies over brown rice, or an occasional grilled chicken breast.

Most nights I snacked on a large bowl of popcorn popped in olive oil. I was eating a low-fat, high-carbohydrate diet. But because the carbs were not refined, for the most part, I thought I was a healthy eater. And not until I hit my forties did anything change.

But boy, did things change. Soon after my fortieth birthday, I noticed my energy level was beginning to wane. By late afternoon I was exhausted. Even if I caught an afternoon nap, I couldn't stay awake much past 9:00 p.m.—and I'd still sleep until 6:30 or 7:00 a.m. I used to be very energetic with only six or seven hours' sleep. What happened?

Worst of all for me, I began to gain weight that exercise simply would not do away with. It was just a pound or so a year, but it was beginning to add up. With my strict eating and exercise habits, I could not fathom why this was happening, so I chalked it up to perimenopause.

Ultimately, though, it ticked me off. Why should I lose my vibrancy and vitality in middle age? And if I was consistently gaining a pound or so a year, where would I be in ten years?

HITTING THE BOOKS

I began to research. I read dozens of the newer studies on weight gain and effective exercise. I learned I could be exercising more efficiently so as not to require forty-five minutes of cardio a day. I followed the expert recommendations and began keeping a food journal for the first time in my life, measuring my food to accurately identify the calories in everything I ate. I was shocked. I had thought I was eating around 1,500 calories a day when I was actually eating about 2,600 calories per day! My idea of a proper portion was all out of whack, just like most Americans'.

Once I discovered I was simply eating too many calories, I thought the solution would also be simple: eat less of what I was eating! The problem was, I was left unsatiated. It seemed I was *always* hungry. And I was still very fatigued.

I was unwilling to use diet or appetite-suppressant pills because I never liked their side effects, so I went back to research more about hunger and appetite. Why

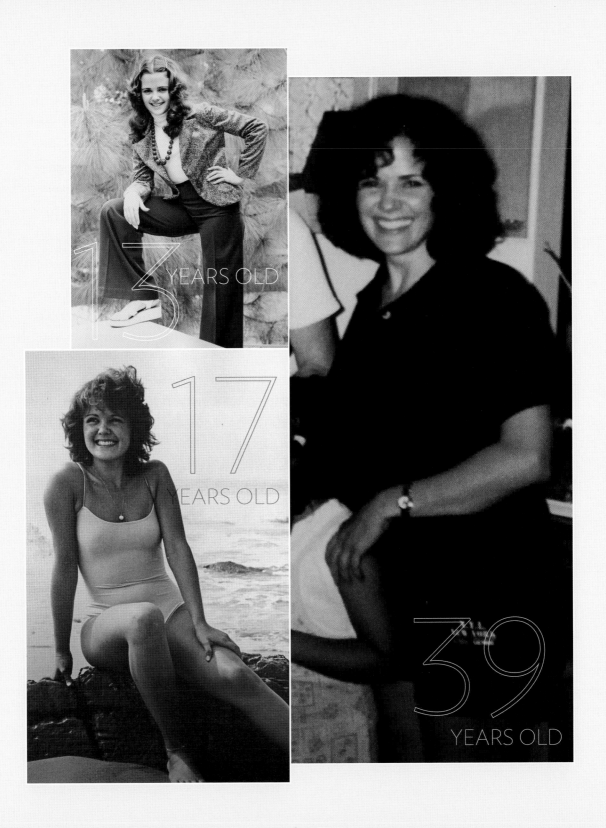

13 YEARS OLD

17 YEARS OLD

39 YEARS OLD

was I so hungry all the time? That was my problem. I was convinced that no human can walk around hungry and deprived for any length of time without satisfying that hunger. Certainly, I couldn't. There must be another answer.

I began analyzing the composition of the foods I was eating and the effect they had on my body. When I broke them down to basics, I learned that carbohydrates are metabolized as sugar, giving a quick energy rise and subsequent fall. Proteins stabilize blood sugar levels. Fats help us to absorb nutrients and also provide that all-important satiety factor.

With that, I now focused on what I was eating at each meal, how it was affecting my energy level, and whether it was keeping hunger at bay. I found that my "healthy" breakfast of a bran muffin or a whole-wheat bagel was mainly carbs with a bit of fat. There was almost no protein. I found my lunches of fruit and yogurt or a salad with a slice of whole-wheat toast were also mainly carbs with a little fat and, again, almost no protein. Dinner was the same; all my favorite foods—salads, baked potatoes, pasta, veggies, and rice—were carb-heavy with just a little bit of fat.

My diet was essentially 70 percent carbs, 15 percent protein, and 15 percent fat. No wonder I was tired—I was giving my body a rush of energy from carbohydrates, and without enough protein to stabilize my blood sugar, I was crashing. To top it off, I wasn't eating enough fat to remain satiated, so I was eating more calories than I needed.

REVAMPING THE EATING PLAN

To alter my meals, I started with breakfast. I relinquished my muffin or bagel and substituted a piece of whole-grain toast with an egg and a slice of cheese. I wasn't full. The next day, I decided to dump the slice of cheese and add another egg and put it on half of a whole-wheat bagel. I found I had great energy and wasn't hungry for about four hours. Bingo.

Lunch was next. I learned about the glycemic index of foods—the higher the sugar/starch content, the higher the food rates on the glycemic index and the more your body will react to that food by gaining quick energy followed by a crash. Vegetables, particularly the non-starchy ones like broccoli, peppers, and tomatoes, are generally much lower on the glycemic index than fruits, which have a lot of natural sugar. So I decided to forgo fruit at lunch and substitute sliced tomatoes and cucumbers with seasoned salt, then eat a large chicken breast or an open-faced sandwich with a protein, such as tuna or turkey with cheese. Once again, my energy level remained high, and I was not hungry until dinner.

For dinner, I continued my lifelong habit of starting with a huge salad. I just made sure to use the lower-glycemic veggies in it, such as red and green cabbage, broccoli, and cucumber, and I cut back on some of the higher-glycemic carrots, using just one or two. Instead of a carb-heavy entrée, like a large baked potato or pasta with white sauce, I tried rotisserie chicken or salmon. I quickly found I could add some starch to my dinner, like half a cup of brown rice or half of a baked potato, and I still had high energy.

Now that I had revamped my ratios of carbs/protein/fat at each meal to roughly 40 percent carbs, 30 percent protein, and 30 percent fat, give or take a bit, it was actually *easy* for me to reduce my daily calorie intake to 1,700 to 1,800 calories per day. Allocated loosely in this ratio, that number of calories completely satisfied me. In fact, it was hard for me to believe that I was eating fewer calories than I used to, because the constant hunger was gone.

EUREKA—SUCCESS!

It took only about two days of eating this way to convince me to keep with it. Almost immediately, my insatiable hunger and debilitating late-afternoon fatigue vanished.

Within a week or so, the scale was starting to move down—from 113.9 pounds to 112 pounds. After four weeks, I was at 110.5 pounds. After another four weeks, I was at 108.9 pounds. A few weeks after that, I hit 107.2 pounds. I've maintained my weight at 107 to 108 pounds effortlessly ever since.

I had found the perfect eating plan and the secret to exercising efficiently, enabling me to cut almost in half the time I was devoting to exercise (and I give you these secrets in Part III, Revamp the Way You're Exercising). But I knew from my past experience, and the experience of millions of others, that that was only half the battle. The next trick was figuring out how to maintain this winning combination forever. I wanted off the diet roller coaster for good. I began asking myself, "What is one of the main reasons dieters fall off the wagon, time and time again?" And the answer became obvious: stress.

Interestingly, by the time I found the magic eating and exercise bullets, I had come to a point in my life where I had become a pro at managing stress. Despite the many hats I wore as a lawyer, entrepreneur, business owner, wife, and mother, I had learned how to keep my stress levels at a minimum. This, in turn, had the fortuitous side effect of eradicating those cravings to continually binge that used to knock me off every diet I tried. Eureka! Now that I had identified that one remaining component for reaching a balance, my mission was accomplished. I had uncovered the hidden formula to maintain my physical, mental, and spiritual well-being for life.

My energy level is now back to where it was more than a decade ago—I can go to bed at 11:30 p.m. and get up at 6:30 a.m. and have boundless energy throughout the day.

For the first time in my life, I am off the weight-gain/weight-loss seesaw. Weight control no longer runs my life or dominates my thoughts. There is no more struggle and strain, or that uncomfortable feeling of swimming upstream. And I don't feel hungry anymore.

The sense of relief I gained from a simple and healthy weight-control method is immeasurable. The sense of confidence I have enjoyed from this has, in turn, positively enhanced every aspect of my life.

In retrospect, I can see this struggle really wasn't about weight control. It was, and is, about freedom. I found that, like most of us, until I was released from the constant preoccupation with my weight, I was not free to fully participate joyfully in life. I have learned I am not unique in feeling this way.

A REALISTIC, NO-NONSENSE PLAN FOR WEIGHT LOSS

My weight-loss and fitness plan is like no other. It is the culmination of my lifelong struggle to find the weight-loss and exercise techniques that would give me the body I desired. I wanted to look great, feel strong, and have the energy to enjoy the life I am so fortunate to have. I'm happy to say that after thirty years of searching,

I've succeeded.

What makes this plan unique? It takes well-established weight-loss principles and exercise methods and combines them with time-tested stress-management techniques—creating the most potent permanent weight-loss blueprint you'll ever find.

In this book, I'll walk you through my powerful three-part strategy, which begins where all weight loss should—with your mind—and continues to places that others don't, like stress-management training. Then we'll quickly and easily proceed to the specific dietary changes that melt pounds, and the exercise principles that will remold your body to the shape you've always wanted.

So what is the secret? It's in the power of balancing three core components: stress, diet, and exercise. These three critical parts must harmonize, and when they do—wow! Your body will mold into a form you have only dreamed of. And people will notice.

YOUR MIND: THE ULTIMATE SMOKE-AND-MIRRORS MACHINE

Left to its own devices, the body is a machine with a mathematical weight-control system: Calories taken in must equal calories expended. Take in more calories than you expend, and you gain weight. Expend, or burn, more than you take in, and you lose weight.

The formula for weight control is easy, so why do we constantly struggle with those unwanted pounds? If it were really just a matter of taking in the proper number of calories to balance our activity level, you wouldn't have this book in your hands right now. But weight loss isn't really a battle with the body; it's a battle with the mind. And I can help you win that battle.

FOOD ON THE BRAIN

You already know that food is so much more than fuel. It represents comfort. It is a social lubricant and a reward for good behavior. Our culture ladles on the food at every event. Most of us wouldn't think of attending a sporting event without visiting the concession stand. A movie isn't a movie without the popcorn and soda. Break up with your boyfriend? Bring out the ice cream. Something wonderful happens? Bake a cake! We meet up with friends for breakfast, lunch, dinner, or a midafternoon latte. Food is ever-present. How can we not partake? I recently attended a children's soccer match and was shocked when the referee stopped the game thirty minutes into play . . . *for a snack break.*

But here's the rub. Even a small indulgence carries a big potential penalty. Did you know a mere 100 extra calories each day brings you ten extra pounds in a year? And who notices an extra 100 or 200 calories? That's a tiny amount of food—one slice of bread or a cluster of grapes will do it.

In addition, the foods we eat affect our blood sugar levels, which impact appetite. Research into how our hormones affect our weight has helped me understand that permanent weight loss must include stress-management tools. Why? Because stress hormones cause a very real physical craving for high-fat, high-sugar, and high-sodium foods—all those high-calorie, low-nutrient snacks that sabotage our best efforts to live more healthfully.

Old habits die hard. It's no fun at all to rewire our brains to follow a new path, so our minds give us excuses to push back against change. "Your metabolism is sluggish," you tell yourself. "It's genetic," your brain says. "You inherited it from your dad." Or, "It's inevitable at your age to gain a few pounds." All these excuses just keep you from making the changes that could alter everything.

IN SEARCH OF A MAGIC PILL

Perhaps the most dangerous lie your brain tells you is the "magic pill" story. Many of us harbor the delusion that there must be some trick to losing weight, some magic potion that will melt the pounds away once we discover it. No exercise, no change in diet, no alterations to our existing lifestyles necessary—just take the potion, or pill, and poof! The pounds will mystically disappear. Even the savviest among us falls prey to this line of thinking, and marketers know it.

A multibillion-dollar industry is devoted to magic bullets that promise to help us quickly shed pounds and erase the consequences of out-of-control stress, poor eating habits, and sedentary lifestyles. Even when we know it can't be true, thousands of us hand over our hard-earned dollars for that next elixir, wasting years and money.

I did it, too, for thirty years. And it didn't work. But along the way, I finally discovered a simple, straightforward stress-management, eating, and fitness formula that actually worked. And it didn't cost me an arm and a leg. I didn't have to trek into the Andes for exotic ingredients. I didn't have to live at the gym or camp out in the kitchen whipping up flavorless, complicated recipes. And neither do you.

My plan is not a magic bullet. It's just a reasonable, straightforward way of living that is consistently effective for average people who have busy schedules to juggle, don't need another impossible task to add to their already hectic lives, and are no longer willing to be ravenous in exchange for being slim. Listen, I am a wife, mother, lawyer, business owner, healthy lifestyle expert, and writer. If it isn't simple, quick, and straightforward, I don't have time for it. If that sounds like you, then this is your plan.

Take the steps presented in this book in order. They will allow you to find equilibrium in your life and with your weight. I know you want to jump on a weight-loss regime that delivers instantaneous results. I've been there. But if your life is out of balance, you'll never get your weight in balance. The imbalance will be reflected in your body. There is no magic pill. And that's why diets cannot work in the long term. Once you go back to your previous, imbalanced diet and exercise, the weight will return.

Of course, a multitude of additional benefits come from keeping a balance as well, and that is why mine is a lifestyle plan rather than just a weight-loss program.

If I had known years ago what I know now, I first would have addressed the imbalances in my life—the factors causing me unmitigated stress—before I attempted to alter how I was eating and exercising. Had I done so, I would have found both my mind and my body much more receptive to the diet and exercise changes that were required to finally get the results I had been seeking for decades. Knowing this, we'll start by addressing stress management, then proceed to dietary changes, then go on to what I have discovered to be the most effective and efficient ways to exercise.

You can benefit from my mistakes as well as my successes. There have been lots of false starts and wrong turns in my path, and I can help you steer around them, shooting straight toward your goal.

Just follow me.

PART ONE

STRESS LESS TO WEIGH LESS

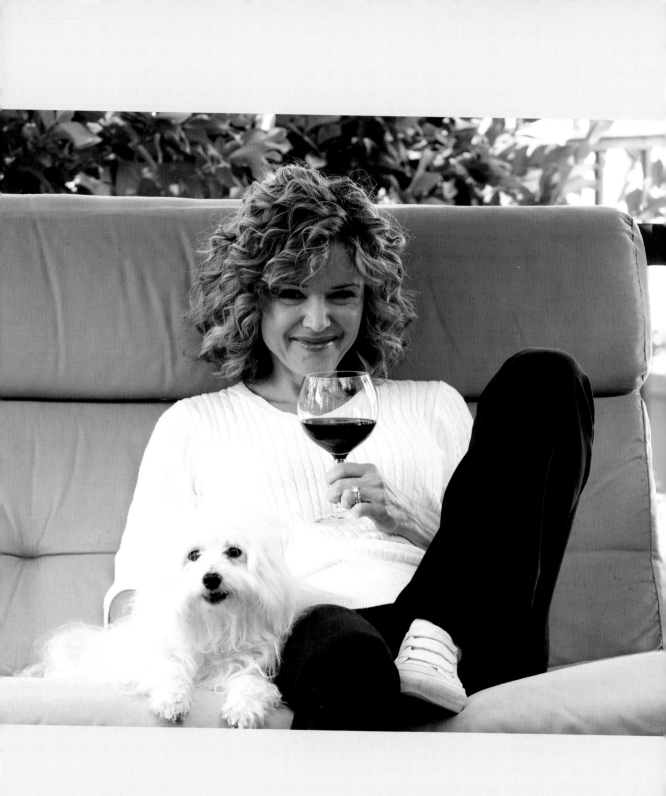

CHAPTER 1

DISCIPLINE YOUR MIND TO RELIEVE YOUR STRESS

Stress has a huge impact on our quality of life as well as our appetites. Until we get our stress under control, even the best weight-loss plans fail. Why? Because, as we have already learned, one of the ways the body reacts to stress is by secreting an overabundance of stress hormones, including cortisol. Cortisol causes physiological cravings as the body seeks comfort through food. That is why we tend to stay on "diets" for only a few months, then fail. It is not that we are simply weak-minded or lack willpower. Under the constant onslaught of overabundant stress hormones, our bodies push us to eat foods that counterbalance the effects of these stress hormones coursing through us. Research has found that most people's stress-induced cravings are for certain foods: high-fat, high-sodium, high-sugar foods—the worst foods for dieters!

So until we learn to manage stress, and thereby avert the dump of excess cortisol into our bodies, we will remain caught in the never-ending cycle of yo-yo dieting. How many times have we jumped from diet to diet, only to fall off the wagon and regain the weight? Not only does the saying "stress kills" relate to physical maladies; stress literally kills our ability to modify our eating.

I have found after years of study and experimentation that the secret to real weight loss, *permanent* weight loss, is to first get stress under control.

I FOUND PRACTICAL TOOLS TO **CONTROL STRESS**, AND YOU CAN TOO

You see the images of me now, as I live today. But there was a time when it strained me to even come out of my bedroom, I was so depleted and depressed.

Well over a decade ago, I was divorced from my kids' father and had been remarried for several years. I had two children, and my new husband, Rob, who was also a lawyer, had two children. We were trying to "blend."

We thought our love would conquer all. Boy, were we in for a wake-up call. It was going to take a lot more than our love if we were to have any shot at etching out a cohesive family and happy marriage with the endless onslaught that came our way from seemingly every direction. If something could go wrong, it did. We had issues with ex-spouses, insomnia-inducing money worries, health concerns, and kids with everything from ADHD to oppositional defiant disorder. I was gaining weight and losing energy to the point where no matter how many hours I slept at night, I needed a nap in the afternoon. And even then the fatigue did not leave me. I was in a black hole of depression. I couldn't imagine what I would be like at age fifty; I was already old and falling apart before age forty.

A WAKE-UP CALL FROM A FRIEND

It was at this point that my dear friend Bob, another lawyer we shared office space with, marched into my office one day to find me with my head on my desk, staring at the wall. "The reason you are depressed," Bob said, "is because you are thinking all the time about what has gone wrong in your life. But there are still a lot of things going right. You still have your husband. You still have your home. You still have this office . . ."

I remember raising my head and staring at him. By God, he was right. I still have hundreds—no, thousands—of things going right in my life, but 99.9 percent of my thoughts were on the few dozen things going wrong. I am not downplaying those things. By all standards, they were very significant, and society would say I was justified in my depressed reaction. But what good was that doing me?

This was the "aha" moment. Bob's words pierced that doom and gloom that I now saw I was creating by my habit of dwelling on the very things I hated most about my existence at that time.

THE LIST OF POSITIVES BEGAN A NEW LIFE

I got out a notepad and started to write. I listed the things going right in my life—from basic things we take for granted to the little things that make life fun. "I can see!" I wrote. "I can walk!" I can breathe, talk, and, more important, *choose what I want to think about*! And that was the key that opened the door to untold joys. Who would've known?

I don't know why we humans tend to dwell on the negative. It's that train-wreck mentality—too horrible not to look. But I now know this: Negative thoughts breed negative thoughts. I proved it.

That day, that list, was the beginning of me pulling out of my dark depression. I kept that baby with me at all times, treating it as precious cargo. Every time I found myself dwelling on the negative, out came the list, and I would gently prod my attention toward the positive.

THE NEW HABIT CREATED AN EXCITING FUTURE

It soon became a habit. When something would go wrong—and plenty of things still did—instead of surrendering myself to the negative stream of thoughts trying to flood in, I used this proactive tool to take control of my state of mind.

It was just the start. The list was an easy, straightforward method of relief that not only taught me the importance of learning how to discipline my thoughts, but also gave me the sweet taste of the peace that follows. And I wanted more.

So began my mission to find other methods and tools to assist me in my quest to master my thoughts. Even the smallest of efforts in this direction brought a greater measure of peace and calm, so it was obvious to me that this path was the one to travel.

And travel I did. I became a stress-tool junkie, loading up on all manner of methods like a beauty junkie fills drawers with hundreds of cosmetics. Anything that came to my attention was worthy of at least inquiry, if not wholesale diving in. I read books, listened to tapes, attended dozens and dozens of weekend retreats, and even spent many full weeks with various teachers who all had wisdom to share with me. I found that there were always at least some nuggets of value I could distill, even if the full program or technique was a turnoff. There was no need to add more stress by trying to pound my square peg into a round hole!

UNTOLD REWARDS FLOW FROM DISCIPLINING OUR THOUGHTS

Distilling all these experiences into one most potent nugget, I learned that the key to a stress-free life is *self-discipline*. Particularly, self-discipline of our thoughts. That is the foundation. No ifs, ands, or buts. There is no freedom from stress without it, and there is no substitute for developing it. But once you do develop it, you will experience an empowerment and enlivened freedom unlike any temporary pleasure you have ever enjoyed before. And all the tools I will give you here are designed to do just that—to aid you in developing discipline over your thoughts. Because that is the key to realizing your dreams. Your thoughts will determine your future.

Why do people put off developing self-discipline? Because they overestimate the work involved to develop it and underestimate the rewards it brings. Before I developed the self-discipline to start governing my thoughts, I was trapped by my old patterns of thought, which brought with them those nasty habits that kept me imprisoned in a body that wasn't serving me as I wanted and a life that did not please me at all.

We have a *right* to live the way we want. We have a right to choose our own goals. We have a right to decide how we want our bodies to look and feel, but unfortunately we do not exercise these rights. Instead, we tend to drift along, victims of our own ignorance of the fact that we can have what we want, if we are willing to take that first step toward developing the self-discipline to govern our thoughts.

RELIEF COMES QUICKER THAN YOU MIGHT THINK

This is not a long process! I started to feel better and happier after taking my very first baby step toward actively governing my thoughts shortly after I turned forty. I understand your reluctance to try it—this was not easy for me to do at the time, either. It seemed like just about everything that could possibly go wrong in my life had done so, or had gone completely sideways, and I was so depleted and dejected, it took what felt like a Herculean effort to just take that first step.

But I didn't have anyone to look to for practical tools. And I needed tools—tools designed to aid a typical person like me: a mom, stepmom, and wife, with a high-pressure job and more demands than I could possibly fulfill. Even though I knew how to meditate and had had a meditation practice for years, it wasn't enough on its own to pull me out of my black hole. Advice to "think positive thoughts" didn't come close to cutting it for me. How the heck do you do that when you have a kid screaming in your face, your financial obligations are beyond your ability to meet them, and you don't have the energy to fight with everyone and still work and earn an income? And just forget about having health and vitality, much less a body and weight you are comfortable with. That was me.

I figured it out so you don't have to. You've got my blueprint. You are holding my private manual. Just take that first step to use one of the tools below that appeals to you. No beating yourself up. That's not allowed. Be patient with yourself. It took you years to form the bad habits of thought that you no longer want. It will take a little time to form new and better ones. But I promise you this: Even a slight move in this direction will bring you some peace. The more effort you apply to it, the faster you'll find your bliss, but you'll experience rewards immediately.

Perfection of effort is not required, by the way. It is the *consistency of attempting* to work these tools that brings the progress. It's like anything else. If I want to tone muscle, lifting a ten-pound weight a few times every day will move me toward my goal much quicker than hoisting a fifty-pound barbell once a week. Yes, it really is true: "Slow and steady wins the race." Just try a little, every day. You'll see.

YOUR STRESS-REDUCTION TOOL KIT

Over the past decades, I've assembled stress-reduction tools that average people can use easily to find relief. I stayed away from the exotic (vacation by private jet to Fiji) in favor of practicality. If it's not practical, then I've found I just won't do it. It has to fit easily into my life. For example, if the dog just threw up, I'm on deadline for work, I've got a stack of bills needing to get paid, and one of the kids just called with a dental emergency (a typical day in my family), what is available to me right now to reduce my stress? Although different people find different things effective for relieving stress, I will share the specific tools that consistently work for me and my family, friends, and clients. I found that once my stress was managed, the repeated, sabotaging cravings disappeared, allowing me to sensibly eat the regular foods I love, which in turn handed me the body I always dreamed of. So let's take a look at this enemy so we can understand it and get it under control.

What is stress? It varies from person to person, but it's essentially tension—that feeling of tightness in the stomach or chest that arises in response to some outer stimulus or even just a thought. It has its place. We need a certain amount of stress to motivate us to move forward in life. It's natural to experience tension when we expose ourselves to new things and experiences.

The problem comes when we have no means of releasing that tension, which puts us in a nearly constant state of mental strain. Stress is cumulative. It's not just a passing feeling; the effects build up. As stress builds, the effects are stored in our bodies. Not only does your appetite spike, but your immune system is suppressed, leaving you vulnerable to more illnesses. Your sleep suffers. It becomes a domino effect, as poor sleep also suppresses the immune system and spikes your appetite. Studies show that those who sleep fewer than seven or eight hours a night tend to weigh more than those who get sufficient rest, and that lack of sleep not only triggers the appetite, but also it increases our desire for high-fat, high-carbohydrate, calorie-dense food.[3]

OPT OUT AS A LIFESTYLE

Before we get to specific stress-management tools, let's address an issue that I consider to be a serious barrier to permanent weight loss and a major dysfunction of American culture: overscheduling. No matter how many stress-management tools you have at your disposal, I have learned they do not compensate for a schedule with too many things to do and not enough time in which to do them.

If you chronically schedule too many activities in your typical day and you're too busy to take a little downtime for yourself, employing stress-management techniques will not ameliorate the stress. You will constantly be battling an appetite brought on by the stress hormones. That's what happened to me.

What to do? "Opt out" as a lifestyle. Don't do things just because everyone else is doing them. Evaluate activities, choose what works for your life, and do only those things. Learn to say no to demands, requests, invitations, and activities that leave

---

3   The specific reason that lack of sleep causes weight gain is because it disrupts two of the hormones associated with regulating appetite (leptin and ghrelin) and also increases the production of cortisol, which is associated with weight gain and belly fat. Results are from a University of Chicago study by Eve Van Cauter, published in *Annals of Internal Medicine*, December 7, 2004.

you with no time for yourself. Until I learned to say no—and mean it—I was always overloaded by stress. You may feel guilty and selfish at first for guarding your downtime, but you'll soon find that you are a much nicer, more present, more productive person in each instance where you choose to commit and say yes. You'll bring a greater benefit to yourself and others when you are not constantly operating from a state of depletion.

With those lessons learned, I now build space into my daily schedule. Without space in my day, I'm going to be stressed, no matter how wonderful the things are that occupy my time and energy. Our culture encourages us to plan every moment and fill our schedules with one activity and obligation after the next, with no time to just be. But the human body and mind require downtime to rejuvenate. I have found my greatest moments of joy and peace just sitting in silence, and then I take that joy and peace with me out into the world.

When I take a break, even just a brief one, the creative energy flows in. Only then do I have anything of value to share with others. Once I recognized this, I stopped feeling guilty about taking time for myself. Taking that time took the form of saying no to some requests and invitations, which felt awful at first. I felt like such a loser! "No, thank you for asking, but I can't attend that event . . . "

But that feeling of being a loser gradually disappeared when I saw that I was being re-formed as a human being. With space in my day, I had plenty of love and compassion to offer others, and that nasty tension that makes us want to do things like blast our horns at rude drivers just faded away.

Saying no can be uncomfortable, especially when you're not used to it. You'll hem and haw and circle around it, perhaps even offering a weak "maybe." That's a big mistake. It works best to just be out with it. Offering excuses and reasons why you can't do something only muddies things and serves as an opening for negotiation. The most important reason for your "no" is that you need your downtime so you won't behave like a jerk because you're depleted. And you don't want to battle an appetite spiked by the stress of overcommitment. But that's your secret; others don't need that information. So just smile, say no, thank you, and keep moving.

Opting out as a lifestyle is the first and most important stress-management tool you need. Once your schedule is under control—and by that, I mean once there is enough space in your day that you aren't rushing from one activity and obligation to the next—then I suggest employing any or all of the tools in the next chapters to actively create a peaceful, productive state of mind—one that is not overrun by the stress hormones.

I list a multitude of tools I use or have found value in at one time or another. You may notice that some of them overlap. Why include the redundancy? Because sometimes just a slight twist on a tool or concept makes it more accessible to me. It all depends on the specific scenario I'm facing. I bet it will be the same for you. If you become familiar with all of them, you'll have a solid library of choices at your disposal when trouble comes a-knockin'.

You'll probably settle on a few staples that click with you. Be proactive with them. Make these choice few a part of your daily life to maintain a basic state of equilibrium at all times. If you commit to that, you'll find "crushing blows" a thing of the past. For me, daily meditation and pranayama (or focused breathing) are non-negotiable. Without them, I spaz. Then I just select from other techniques, should the need arise.

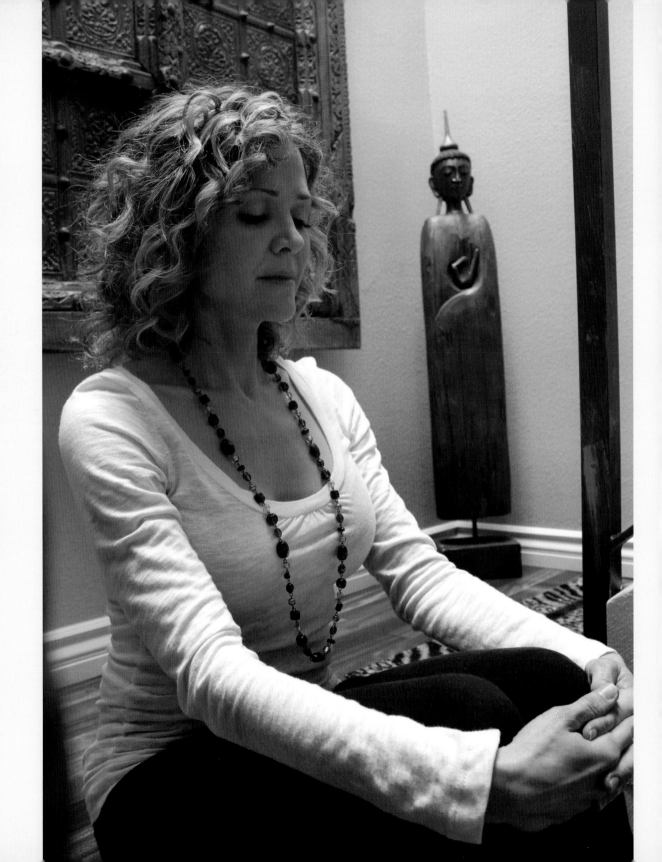

CHAPTER 2

EXPLORE THE MIND-BODY CONNECTION

We've all heard about the "mind-body" connection, but I didn't fully appreciate just how potent a link it was until I experienced how my mind, boiling over with negative thoughts, impulses, complaints, and nagging, was destroying the vitality and health of my body. My negative thoughts added to the mountain of stress I was carrying like a backpack filled with rocks, sending me into regular feeding frenzies on cookies, cakes, and pizza, and ushering my weight along a steady uphill ascent as I entered middle age.

I didn't initially work on modifying my thoughts and reducing my stress as a way to lose weight. At that point in my life, my weight was an annoyance, but far from the worst of my problems. My most immediate and debilitating problem was the overwhelming fatigue that kept me in bed many hours of each day. At the time, I didn't know this exhaustion was one of the effects of depression, which was another consequence of the constant onslaught of negative thoughts circulating in my mind. In my efforts to remedy this mental negativity, my main goal was just to get some relief from that black cloud of doom and weariness that was with me at every waking moment.

It was after I first began to uplift my thoughts a bit—a little while after that "aha" moment with Bob in my office when I began keeping a "list of positives"—that my cravings for junk food started to dissipate. I did not connect the two at that time. First, I simply noticed that I could raise my head off my desk, and I didn't need to sleep so much. It took a while before I realized that in addition to my improved energy level, there was a direct correlation between chewing on mental garbage and putting garbage in my mouth—another one of those "aha" moments.

As I continued to seek out tools to relieve my stress and elevate my mind, I found a double benefit: happier mood and fewer cravings. These improvements set the stage for a body overhaul I never could have foreseen. I realized an important sequence of events had occurred: I had arrived at a more peaceful, less stressed state of mind *before* the excess weight melted off.

And I got more than just a body overhaul—I was gifted with rejuvenation and enrichment in my relationships; a renewed interest in life; an expansive attitude that led me to try new activities like boxing (of all things); and inspiration to get creative in my kitchen for the first time in my life, making mealtime fun by creating easy, low-calorie recipes using all my favorite foods.

Let me walk you through the realizations, tools, and techniques that led me there.

FOUR-COUNT BREATH

The Four-Count Breath is by far the quickest, most practical, and most effective stress reducer. All you do is consciously focus on the breath. You can do it anytime, anywhere, and no one even needs to know. I learned about the calming effects of focused breathing through yoga, but you need not do yoga to benefit from it.

Focused breathing as a relaxation tool is nothing new. It wasn't even new back in the late 1960s when Herbert Benson, M.D., an associate professor of medicine at Harvard Medical School and founder of the Benson-Henry Institute for Mind Body Medicine in Massachusetts, began some groundbreaking research on the mind-body connection and the harmful effects of stress. Among other things, he found that merely focusing on the breath going in and out of the body, with an intention to avoid distracting thoughts, could evoke what he called "The Relaxation Response." And that became the title of his 1975 best-selling book.

I distilled some of Dr. Benson's principles and others I learned through yoga, and that's how I came up with the Four-Count Breath technique. It's simple. Breathe in through your nose while slowly counting to four, then exhale through your nose to the count of four. Focus on the breath with your mind. Listen to the sound of it. If possible, close your eyes. Let the breath be smooth, with no gasping or catching, kind of like a wave flowing in and then drifting away from the shore.

After just three or four of these breaths, you will begin to notice a difference. After you start to feel the evenness in your breath, you can add brief breath retention. Inhale to the count of four, then retain the breath in for a count of one or two seconds. Exhale to the count of four, then retain the breath out for one or two counts. Stop if you feel any difficulty. If retention enhances your stress relief, you can slowly increase the duration.

I find breath retention extremely relaxing. I start by retaining the breath for a single count. Then, slowly, easily, I build the retention to three or four counts, sometimes even six counts or more. If it becomes a struggle, I simply go back to retaining for a single count, or perhaps none.

MAKE FOCUSED BREATHING A GAME

Focused breathing is fun for me. I love playing around with it. When I'm driving and hit a red light, that's a signal to begin the Four-Count Breath. The phone rings? Four-Count Breath starts before I even answer it. The alarm goes off? Four-Count Breath begins. I'm like Pavlov's dog. I've ingrained the habit, so my first response when something stressful happens is to focus on my breath rather than blindly reacting. You can feel the stress just wash away, or at least the worst of it.

Conversely, when I fail to practice the Four-Count Breath in a stressful situation, I can track the dump of cortisol into my system and the cravings that follow. My daughter and I compare notes on this. One day she called me, really upset. Another driver had just turned left in front of her, and my daughter had to swerve hard to avoid an accident. It scared her pretty badly, and instead of immediately turning to the Four-Count Breath, she rolled her window down and screamed at the other driver. A few hours later? Massive binge.

The same thing happens to me, and I'm betting it happens to you. And it doesn't take anything as obvious as a near-accident to evoke this stress response. We experience it many times a day, from a multitude of sources. A tense phone call, a nasty e-mail, a mailbox full of bills, overload at work, and kids' schedules that won't relent . . . In fact, it may not be just one attention-getting event; stress is cumulative, so we collect it and keep adding to our storehouse. No wonder we're ever more vulnerable to supersized meals and unconscious snacking.

The good news? The opposite also is true: We can build a reserve of calm and peace that becomes available for us to draw from, like money in the bank. We can fill our tanks, so to speak, and have that reservoir available. That's what I am doing by using little cues during the day to trigger my Four-Count Breath. I'm making deposits into my calm bank.

FOCUSED BREATHING REDUCES CRAVINGS

I've been practicing focused breathing for several years now, and I see the direct correlation between consistent use of the Four-Count Breath and a big reduction in cravings. When I first started developing my weight-loss plan in the mid-2000s, I was still having a once-a-week pig-out to indulge my appetite. I needed this weekly event to generate the willpower to fight my many cravings. Sometimes it was quite a strain to wait for the weekly pig-out to indulge.

Because I record everything I eat—and have for years—I can track the change in my habits. Even though I still recommend that you have your weekly pig-out, I can see that I no longer do this—not because of iron willpower but because diminished cravings allow me to skip it altogether without missing a thing. What freedom.

Had you told me years ago this would happen, I'd have said you didn't know me at all. Food cravings have been a frustrating part of my life since I was a little girl sneaking after-school Ding Dongs and Hostess Cup Cakes (you know, the chocolate ones with the white squiggled line of icing on top).

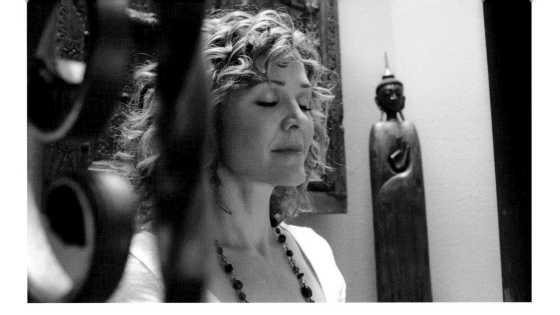

MEDITATION

For many, the word "meditation" conjures up images of people in saffron-colored robes sitting in Lotus pose on stone floors, burning incense and chanting. And there are those who meditate in that manner. But don't let the word and its connotations freak you out and close you off to what it offers.

Multiple studies have found that meditation positively impacts the area of the brain in charge of the autonomic nervous system—the part of our nervous system that controls things like blood pressure, heart rate, digestion, elimination, and the immune system. These are the systems negatively affected by stress. But you can counteract those negative effects with meditation. In short, it calms you, lowering the amount of stress hormones in your system, along with their attendant cravings.

You don't have to learn Eastern philosophy or subscribe to metaphysics to benefit from meditation and its incredible stress-reduction capabilities. According to my Webster's dictionary, to meditate merely means "to engage in contemplation; reflect." Anyone with any set of beliefs—or nonbelief—can benefit. You need simply to be willing to set aside a few minutes to be quiet.

I began meditating when I was in my twenties. This was back in the early '80s, so it wasn't a popular thing to do, and I can no longer recall exactly what prompted me to begin. But the act of sitting quietly with my eyes closed and concentrating on breathing evenly always calmed me, and that felt good.

It didn't take me long to notice that when I engaged in quiet contemplation on a daily basis, it was easier for me to enter that state of bliss we can all find with enough practice and dedication. It opened up a whole new vista for me. I began a deeply personal, lovely journey that continued to expand my internal awareness. I liked having a private way of touching serenity, unrelated to anything occurring "out here." Once you learn to access joy within yourself, independent of the people and circumstances that surround you, you're free. You no longer need so much control over your outer world. It is this surrender of control that gifts us with reduced stress.

HOW DO YOU MEDITATE?

Just as with yoga, a multitude of meditation styles and teachings exist that can lead you in the right direction. You can find a teacher or a school to assist you in learning the techniques, but the core of meditation practice involves simply sitting quietly, finding one thing to focus on, gently prompting your focus back to this one thing when it begins to wander, and then observing how the thoughts slow down and give way to quiet peace.

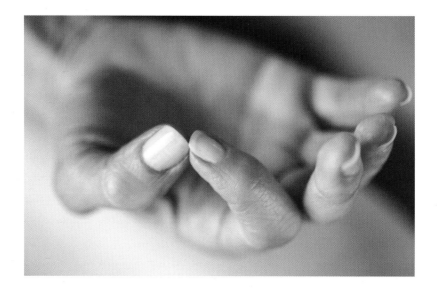

You can focus on anything to begin your meditation—a flower, a sound, a single thought, a word. Anything. I like to begin my meditation practice by reading a bit of something uplifting, ranging from Bible passages to the yoga sutras to Joel Goldsmith's or Wayne Dyer's writings or interpretations of the Tao Te Ching. I'll read anything that expands and elevates my consciousness. I take one statement, or just one word, from my reading and ponder it. Then I focus on my breath. I'll begin the Four-Count Breath (see page 26) and turn my entire focus to it. Just focusing on this measured breathing begins to quiet the jumble of thoughts in my mind.

As your thoughts slow and you become more still, you'll feel your body releasing tension. If you continue, your relaxed state deepens to a sense of peace, later followed by moments of pure bliss. It's the best high ever, and it's legal. And it reduces stress. There is no downside.

CONSISTENCY IS KEY

I think many people forgo meditation, even after learning of its blissful benefits, because they mistakenly believe a regular meditation practice is very time-consuming. It does not have to be. After decades of meditating and studying it with various meditation groups and individual teachers and teachings, I have found that it is the consistency of my practice of meditation, rather than any specific technique or the length of time I spend in meditation, that bestows the core value.

All you need to do is commit to taking a few moments in your day—every day—to sit quietly and find a single-point focus. I have found it immensely helpful to sit in the same spot every day for meditation, if at all possible. That spot becomes a trigger for your mind to slow the thoughts. It becomes a reflex, just like our stomachs are trained to start growling at dinnertime. This slowing of thoughts is the gateway to meditation, a state in which the thoughts slow to a stop (at least at times). When you find that soothing, peaceful space between the thoughts, you will never want to leave. Once you experience that, you'll be hooked, and being consistent with your meditation practice will no longer take any effort at all.

My morning meditation practice is the cornerstone of my life and is nonnegotiable. Even if I have to leave the house at 5:00 a.m., I'll set my alarm a few minutes early to meditate first. Some mornings I devote only five minutes to it (like those days I have to be somewhere at an ungodly hour); other mornings (particularly on the weekends) I have several hours to devote to my practice. More is definitely better, but consistency trumps quantity of time. On the rare occasion that I skip my morning meditation (and if I do, I always do a session later in the day), I have noticed that, generally, the day does not flow as smoothly. It's probably because I didn't center myself in peace before getting banged up by all manner of stuff that waits for each of us right outside the door.

Just as regular exercise is necessary to tone your muscles, it's necessary that you make your meditation practice a regular part of your day to gain the benefit of reduced stress and lower levels of stress hormones, and to increase the joyful quality of your life. You'll find it well worth it.

REGULAR EXERCISE

I've devoted a whole section of this book to exercise (Part III: Revamp the Way You're Exercising), but it's still important to include it here. That's because among its other tremendous benefits, exercise is a natural stress reducer. Exercise reduces physical and emotional tension built up in the body. It does this physically through systems that help your body dispose of excess stress hormones and other by-products of stress. It helps emotionally by triggering the release of endorphins, the "happy" hormones that cause us to feel good.

Studies have confirmed again and again that exercise improves mood, and it does so fairly quickly. You don't need a full hour; just twenty minutes can reduce the production and effects of stress hormones. I've found that if I'm short on time, even a ten-minute walk can significantly reduce any stress I may feel. It's even better if I can take that walk outdoors! (Again, research confirms this; we release more endorphins when we exercise outside.)

When it comes to battling stress levels, you don't have to engage in high-impact cardio exercise to gain significant benefits. You just need to move. Activities like gardening and leisurely swimming are ideal for stress reduction; they both get you moving outside.

The more regular the exercise, the better chance your body has to vent all that built-up tension. If you find something you enjoy doing, you're more likely to be consistent with it. So find several activities you like, and have them at your disposal so you can spring into action if you feel stress building up. Here's what I do. I keep a pair of tennis shoes in the trunk of my car so I can always grab a quick walk if I want to, wherever I am. Walking is my go-to stress-reduction activity of choice. It's easy, it can be done anywhere, and best of all, I can intersperse short bouts of it throughout my day, especially if I'm prepared with my shoes always packed in my car.

I walk and use my cell phone to return calls, especially if I have a stressful call to return. The walking counteracts the stress, and it works particularly well if I walk a few minutes to start revving up the endorphins before I dial.

When I'm waiting at the airport, I walk until boarding time to maintain calmness. I also like to take about a twenty-minute walk first thing in the morning, right before I meditate, as I have found this enhances the depth of my meditations, probably because the short stroll prepares my body and mind to sit in stillness.

When I was in India recently, I was surprised to learn that the people in that country have grave concerns about India becoming the world's number one cardiac disease capital. Why? As Western lifestyle influences have gained traction there, so have our less-desired habits, including crazy scheduling and no downtime, leading to massive stress. This stress is the main culprit behind heart disease. And the recommendation from leading Indian cardiologists? Walk more: intersperse quick little walks every twenty minutes at your desk if you can't fit in a solid thirty or forty minutes at any one time.

Good advice.

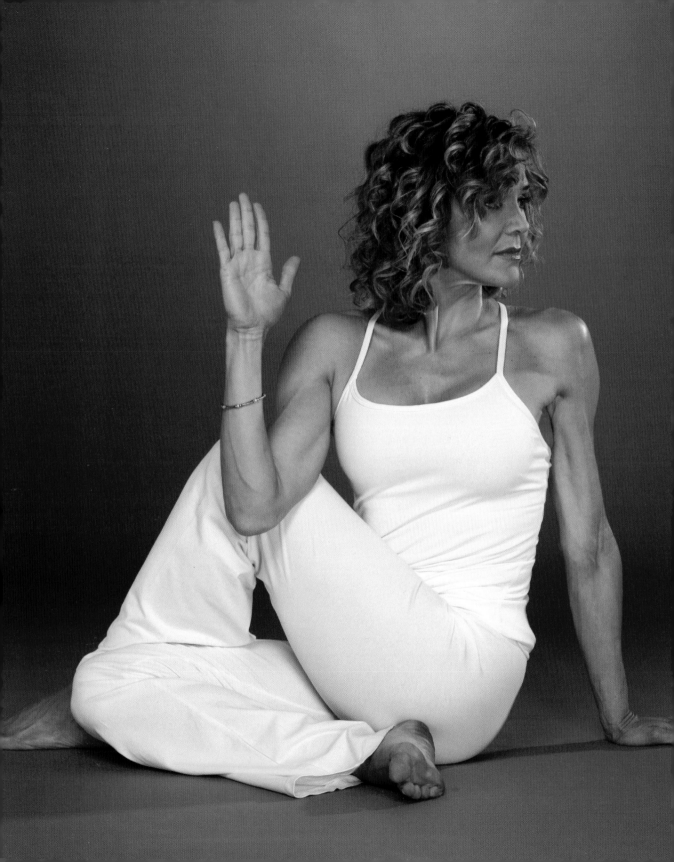

CHAPTER 3

YOGA, THE GREAT STRESS RELIEVER

Although I believe yoga is good for everyone, I understand it's not everyone's cup of tea. But I will say a few things here about how yoga greatly contributes to stress reduction, which, in turn, directly impacts your weight. Before I lose your attention, I'll say right away that although I believe those ninety-minute yoga classes are great, and I personally enjoy them, you can get a lot of yoga's stress-reduction benefits from a ten-minute yoga sequence performed just a couple of times a week. I'll give you some examples later in this chapter.

I did not start yoga until I was forty years old. Over time, it has gifted me with a level of peace I never could have anticipated. With consistent yoga practice, my personality has shifted from a hard-core type A personality to one that is much mellower and filled with a lot less angst. My daughter, although she loves me dearly, gets rather annoyed by this. She complains that her children will never believe I was the tough taskmaster she grew up with. "They'll think Grandma was just a sweet, kind, mellow little lady," she says. I laugh about that, because she's probably right.

As the harsh edges of my personality softened, my body slimmed. I don't believe this was coincidental. I believe (and research backs this up) that the consistent yoga practice reduced my stress levels significantly, which in turn reduced the secretions of stress hormones that used to constantly flood my body, which in turn reduced my cravings and addictions to all those nasty high-fat, high-sugar, and high-sodium foods. Who wouldn't lose weight in this scenario?

Multiple medical studies have confirmed that yoga is one of the premier stress reducers. According to research published by Harvard Medical School in 2009, yoga has been found to slow the heart rate, lower blood pressure, and ease respiration.[4] In short, it decreases stress. Decreased stress means lower levels of stress hormones circulating in your body, which, in turn, cuts cravings. Fewer cravings make weight loss and control a *lot* easier to achieve.

WHAT IS YOGA?

In the Western world, when we hear the word "yoga" we typically think of the physical postures, or asanas, that are associated with it. But yoga is far, far more than that. According to multiple ancient and contemporary writings, yoga means union of the mind, body, and spirit. In the yoga sutras, the ancient Sanskrit texts, yoga is defined as "yogas chitta vritti nirodha"—the stilling of the fluctuations of the mind. This is usually surprising to the Westerner, as we generally see yoga as a physical form of exercise for strength and flexibility. But that is only the outer appearance. The deeper intent of yoga is to still the mind.

I took my first yoga teacher training program in 2008. My first assignment was to answer the question "What is yoga?" I wrote just a phrase: "alignment of the body that coincides with or causes alignment of the mind, creating perfect balance." I completed that program and an additional three hundred hours of training, and that's still what yoga is for me.

---

4   Harvard Medical School, "Yoga for Anxiety and Depression," *Harvard Mental Health Letter*, April 2009.

MY HISTORY WITH YOGA

When I started doing yoga in 2000, I didn't know the first thing about it. I happened into a small class of about six women taught by a lovely young lady named Kinnary Patel. Kinnary was the real deal. She grew up doing yoga as a child in India, and she taught Iyengar-style yoga. Iyengar yoga is named after B.K.S. Iyengar, the renowned yogi in India who runs his own institute and after whom hundreds of Iyengar institutes worldwide are named. Iyengar yoga focuses on very precise alignment in the poses, or asanas.

In hindsight, that precision of alignment and intense attention to detail made it the best way to start learning yoga for me. I stuck with it, because it seemed to me that no matter how rough the class was, I always felt terrific afterwards—physically, emotionally, and spiritually.

After about a year studying Iyengar yoga, I was ready to try something new. I joined a Hatha flow class taught through the emeritus program of our school district, even though I had no idea what it was. The class was held in a portable building at an elementary school—not very yoga-like. But it was about ten dollars per session, so I thought I'd check it out for a semester.

Marlene Geoghan taught the class. She was in her sixties, and she was quiet and stern. But I sensed a wicked sense of humor beneath the surface. After the first night, I was in love. It was a new and exciting way to practice yoga, fast-moving. Instead of assuming a pose and holding it the way I was used to, we "flowed" from one pose to the next, using our breath to carry us into the next asana. I even broke a sweat, which appealed to that Western, athletic side of me.

Marlene was amazing. Despite teaching three classes a night, four days a week—or perhaps because of it—she had incredible vitality. Much of the time, she did most of the class with us. Marlene didn't hesitate to pop up into a perfectly aligned head-stand in the middle of the room, so she inspired us all to break through our natural fears of moving in ways we hadn't since we were kids. Those breakthroughs carried through to everyday life. Once you overcome your fear of turning your body completely upside down, you don't get as worked up over a mishap at the office or a disagreement with your spouse. I saw that yoga was transformative on every level.

After a year, I moved on to Marlene's Ashtanga yoga classes. Ashtanga yoga is a more vigorous, athletic type of yoga. It is the best of the "Vinyasa flow" type of yoga classes, and certainly one of the most fun. Ashtanga yoga comprises six different series of poses. Each series has a set sequence. I started with the primary series and moved on from there.

After several years of Ashtanga practice, my schedule changed pretty dramatically. My husband and I, who were practicing law together in California, were brought in as co-counsel on a medical malpractice case in Arizona. That case led to others, so we took the bar exam and got licensed in Arizona as well. Very quickly, we had a full stable of Arizona cases and began traveling regularly between our California home and Phoenix, Arizona. We set up an office in downtown Phoenix and bought a condo to live in while we were there.

The new commute between Orange County and Phoenix left no time for Marlene. I still miss her and her classes tremendously. She holds a special place in my heart. Yoga teachers are like that. When you find the one for you, they impact you on a multitude of levels. Yoga is like the playground for adults, and Marlene was the coolest older kid who masters the monkey bars before everyone else, then graciously offers instruction so that you, too, can fly.

Now that I didn't have a regular yoga home, I began taking yoga classes all over the place, learning a multitude of styles and bringing facets of all of them into my own practice. I went back to taking Iyengar classes, and I took hundreds of different Vinyasa flow classes from myriad teachers. "Vinyasa" yoga just means a sequence of poses linked together using the breath. So within Vinyasa flow classes, there is an infinite variety of teaching styles and sequences of poses. I liked elements of all of them and found a nice balance by taking all different types of classes.

YOGA TEACHER TRAINING—WHEW!

I had been practicing yoga for about eight years when I decided to participate in my first formal, intense teacher-training program. It was a two-hundred-hour program offered through YogaWorks yoga studio and certified by Yoga Alliance (a non-profit international organization that strives to register both yoga schools and yoga

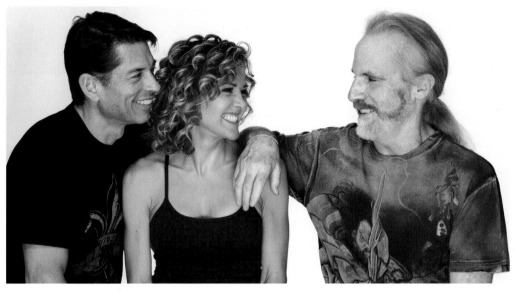

Rob, Holly, and Bob Metzler

teachers who have complied with its standards for instruction). The program took place over three months and included instruction in anatomy, philosophy, and history, as well as the physical poses.

I had no intention of turning my back on my law practice to become a yoga teacher. But by then I had reaped such marked benefits from yoga practice that I wanted to seek a deeper understanding and knowledge of all its aspects. And I knew I'd be compelled at some point to share my experience with others. I wanted the means to effectively convey what I'd learned to others, so they could experience it too.

The training program was brutal but enlightening. And it fundamentally changed me on every level. It's like I had a cellular restructuring of both my mind and body. I felt an incredible sense of emerging mastery of my internal world that coincided with a deep humility and ripening appreciation for all that is.

I finished the program and received a two-hundred-hour Registered Yoga Teacher (RYT) designation by Yoga Alliance. So what did I do with it? I signed up for the next level, this time a three-hundred-hour program that took place over six months. Not only did we receive more instruction in anatomy, philosophy, and history, we also received instruction in injury management and pranayama, the yogic art of breath control believed to balance energy.

In addition to all that instruction, and most valuably, we were paired up with a mentor or master teacher. I apprenticed with Bob Metzler, a handsome, craggy, sea captain–type, with blue eyes and a long silver ponytail, who could either scare the bejesus out of you or, if you got his sense of humor, make you fall in love with him. I "got" Bob. (I admit I was a bit afraid of him at first.) He doesn't suffer fools lightly, although I quickly found he was not annoyed by even ignorant questions if he discerned they were asked sincerely.

Bob is a certified Iyengar teacher who has studied in India and dedicated himself completely to his craft. I reaped the benefit of his piercing insight into yoga as I followed him around like a puppy for six months, taking his classes, assisting his classes, and watching his classes. All this was in addition to the classroom hours required of us and the hours spent observing other instructors and sitting in on their classes to round out our experience. In addition to Bob's formal mentorship, he graciously met me at Starbucks time and again, for hours at a time, to answer my never-ending questions.

Of course, I complained at the time about the intensity of the training and the demands made on us students. It was exhausting. But once again, I found my awareness of yoga expanded and realized that I had barely scratched the surface of what yoga had to offer.

I ADD YOGA TEACHER TO MY RÉSUMÉ

When I completed the training, Yoga Alliance designated me as a five-hundred-hour RYT. I accepted a teaching offer at the YogaWorks studio as well. I taught two of my own weekly classes and filled in for other teachers, both in the Vinyasa flow and Iyengar styles. This forced me to mold my training and experience to benefit disparate groups of students.

The experience taught me to become efficient with yoga, and I found what I believe are the most effective yoga poses for stress management. I call them my Ten-Minute Yoga Sequences. These quick yoga sequences are fantastic stress reducers, and I highly recommend them for those who don't have time for a full sixty- to ninety-minute yoga class.

TEN-MINUTE YOGA SEQUENCES

I feel best when I take two full yoga classes a week (as well as my other exercise, which is described in Part III, Revamp the Way You're Exercising). But during weeks I can't make it to my regular yoga classes, I do these quick Ten-Minute Yoga Sequences about four days a week. The Ten-Minute Yoga Sequences are specifically designed to reduce stress and restore equanimity.

I learned from my teacher training that specific sequencing of poses can create a specific effect. If you are tired and want more vigor, a sequence focused on backbends of all sorts will energize you. If you are feeling down or depressed, chest-opening poses help to heal the heart and elevate mood. If you are emotionally drained, twists "squeeze" out the emotion, much like twisting a wet rag squeezes out the liquid. If you have back pain, hip pain, shoulder pain—any kind of pain—certain asanas are better than others for healing.

For all of these needs, there is an infinite variety of poses, classes, and teachers to lead you in the right direction. But for use as one of our stress-reduction tools, I follow the well-known "Inversions, Backbends, Twists" sequencing in my Ten-Minute Yoga Sequences.

That might sound weird to those who are unfamiliar with yoga, so allow me to explain the formula. I have found that the quickest, most effective yoga sequence for stress relief is an inversion (position in which your head is below the level of your heart), a backbend, and then a twist. I learned from my yoga teacher training that backbends should follow inversions, not precede them, and twists are generally good to do toward the end of the practice to neutralize and relieve the spine.

What I also found was that even if I omitted the rest of the yoga sequence (such as the standard standing poses like Triangle, or Trikonasana, and the standard seated poses, such as deep forward folds like Paschimottanasana, also called Extreme Stretch of the West), I still experienced quite a calming effect by doing just one or two inversions, a few backbends, and one twist to each side.

I noticed I got the biggest bang for my buck if I held the inversion for at least three minutes, did a couple of quick backbends, then did a long-hold twist. This pattern didn't give me the same level of stress reduction as a ninety-minute practice, but it came close—and besides, I don't have time to do ninety minutes every day!

So I adopted Ten-Minute Yoga Sequences as my quick antidote for stress. Below, I'll explain how to perform the poses I use in my Ten-Minute Sequences. After I explain how to perform the poses, I will give you an actual Beginner Ten-Minute Yoga Sequence, Intermediate Ten-Minute Yoga Sequence, and Advanced Ten-Minute Yoga Sequence that you can do yourself. Once you get comfortable with the poses and Ten-Minute Yoga Sequences, you can then create your own sequences by choosing from the poses below. Just be sure to choose at least one inversion, one backbend, and one twist.

YOGA POSES FOR
TEN-MINUTE SEQUENCES

The following pages provide an explanation of how to perform the yoga poses I use in my Ten-Minute Sequences. I'll start with poses that beginners can practice safely, then I'll progress to poses that you should do only if you're experienced.

Even if you have the experience, always choose from the beginner's options if you're performing the sequence without warming up. I always do. And by the way, this is far from an exhaustive list of inversions, backbends, and twists. These are merely examples of the ones I tend to use in these short sequences.

Although I enjoy the yoga studio environment, one of the best things about yoga is that you can do it anywhere. You can do it in your home, in the park, on the beach—any space will do. In India, it's often practiced on stone floors without mats.

(Note: Consult your doctor before beginning any exercise program, including yoga. Some of the poses can exacerbate certain physical conditions and illnesses, and should not be practiced. Please consult medical professionals before attempting any of these poses to ensure that you can safely practice them. The best way to safely learn any of these poses is by studying with a well-trained and experienced yoga teacher.)

Let's get started!

Starting pose—Tadasana (Mountain Pose)

Generally, we start most yoga sequences in **Tadasana**, or **Mountain Pose**. Tadasana is a simple standing pose that helps root you in the stability and balance that you bring into the rest of the sequence.

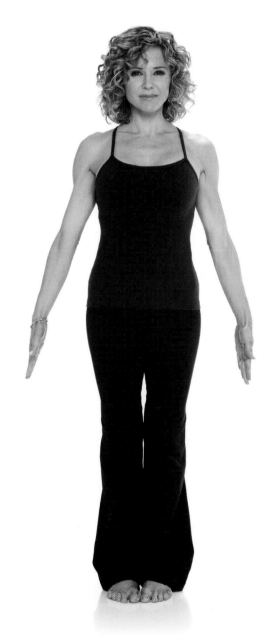

TADASANA (MOUNTAIN POSE): Stand at the front of your mat. Bring your big toes together, with the heels slightly separated. (If this is uncomfortable, you can stand with your feet hip-width apart.) Firm your thighs, and lift the kneecaps. Drop your tailbone toward the floor, as you lift through the crown of your head. Spread your collarbones, and let your shoulder blades descend down your back. Reach your hands down, palms open and facing your thighs, with your arms slightly away from your body. Steady your gaze straight in front of you and take deep, even breaths, inhaling and exhaling through the nose.

Inversions

Any pose in which you bring your head below your heart is called an inversion. For our stress-management purpose here, I include inversions because they tend to calm the mind, but you can reap a host of other benefits from them. Inversions minimize fatigue and increase mental clarity and alertness, for example. They're also considered to be great antiaging tools, as you flip the effect of gravity on your body. There are additional benefits, but those I've just mentioned are reason enough for me to do them regularly. (Note: Many inverted poses should not be practiced

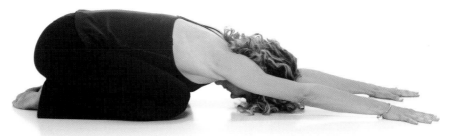

UTTHITA BALASANA (EXTENDED CHILD'S POSE): Kneel on the floor with your knees hip-width apart and big toes touching. Sink your buttocks to your heels and bend your torso over your legs. Reach your arms forward and bring your forehead to the floor.

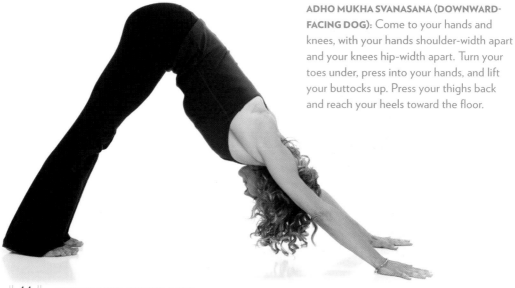

ADHO MUKHA SVANASANA (DOWNWARD-FACING DOG): Come to your hands and knees, with your hands shoulder-width apart and your knees hip-width apart. Turn your toes under, press into your hands, and lift your buttocks up. Press your thighs back and reach your heels toward the floor.

by those with certain health conditions, such as high blood pressure, glaucoma, neck injuries, and others, or during pregnancy or menstruation. Consult your doctor before starting or participating in any exercise program, including yoga.) You can choose any of the inversions that are appropriate and safe for your level of practice to gain the stress-reduction benefit. **Utthita Balasana**, or **Extended Child's Pose,** is a simple inversion that most beginners can practice. The classic **Adho Mukha Svana-sana**, or **Downward-Facing Dog Pose**, is also an inversion. More-advanced inversions involve bringing your feet above your head, such as in **Salamba Sarvangasana**, or **Shoulder Stand**.

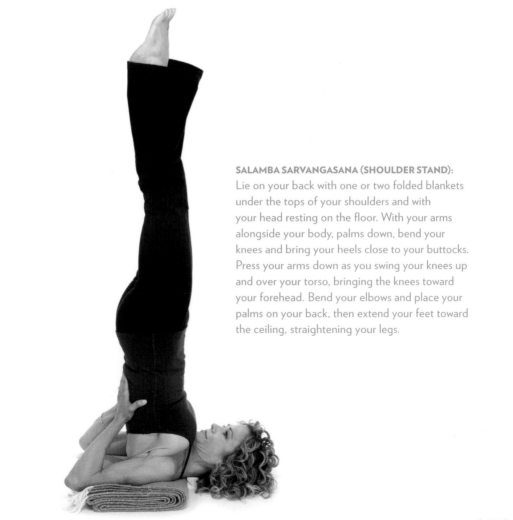

SALAMBA SARVANGASANA (SHOULDER STAND):
Lie on your back with one or two folded blankets under the tops of your shoulders and with your head resting on the floor. With your arms alongside your body, palms down, bend your knees and bring your heels close to your buttocks. Press your arms down as you swing your knees up and over your torso, bringing the knees toward your forehead. Bend your elbows and place your palms on your back, then extend your feet toward the ceiling, straightening your legs.

Adho Mukha Vrksasana, or **Handstand**, is just a heck of a lot of fun. Handstands fill you with a sense of joy and abandon—the same feeling we all used to get when we were out on the playground as kids. When you get into the full pose, there's a sweet spot of full balance, and you feel weightless for a moment. Hitting this sweet spot is always accompanied, for me anyway, by a literal jolt of pure joy that leaves me laughing.

Perhaps the most valuable aspect of Handstand (sometimes called "full arm balance") is that it is the biggest fear-killer of all the asanas. As Bob Metzler told us, "Once you lose your fear of full arm balance, your general level of fear in everyday life has also gone way down." I have certainly found this to be true.

Sirsasana, or **Headstand**, is called the king of asanas, as it is prized as one of the most, if not *the* most, beneficial of all the asanas. One of the main benefits of Headstand is that it can be held much longer than most of the other full inversions, especially if you are supported by a wall. Even if I start my Ten-Minute Yoga Sequence with a couple of quick Handstands (and many times I do, just because it is so darn fun), I usually do Headstand next and hold it for a while. After years of practice, I'm able to hold it for six minutes or more. You should start out slower, beginning with fifteen or twenty seconds and increasing by ten- or fifteen-second increments until you can hold it for at least three minutes. A word of caution: You should do only one Headstand per yoga session to avoid headaches.

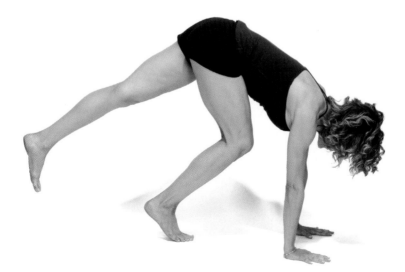

ADHO MUKHA VRKSASANA (HANDSTAND): Start in Downward-Facing Dog with your hands a few inches from a wall. Walk your feet forward until your shoulders are perpendicular to your wrists. Bend one leg under your chest in a lunge position, and raise the other leg to prepare to kick up. Kick up with the bent leg as you swing the raised leg up. Reach both heels to the wall.

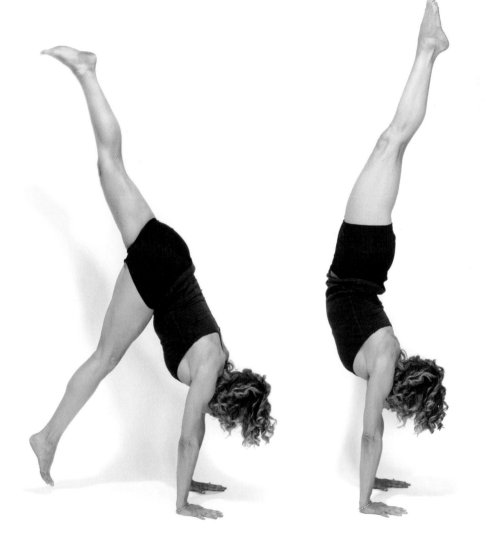

Whenever I do a Headstand, I usually follow it with a Shoulder Stand. This relieves the neck and upper back from Headstand and counterbalances it. (If you're short on time, you can also follow it with Setu Bandha Sarvangasana, or Bridge Pose, explained more fully in the Backbends section. Bridge is a backbend that also counterbalances the Headstand, so it's a great time-saver.)

After doing inversions, I feel lighter and freer for hours afterward. That is why I almost always include full inversions in my yoga practice, and I always include them in these abbreviated ten-minute sessions.

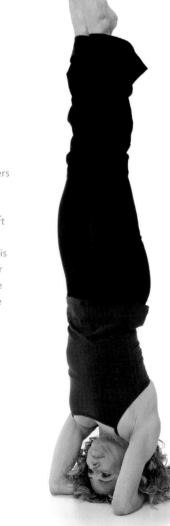

SIRSASANA (HEADSTAND): Come to your hands and knees facing a wall. Bend your arms and bring your elbows to the floor, shoulder-width apart. Interlace your fingers and cup your hands. Place the crown of your head on the floor with your hands lightly cupping the back of your head. Lift your knees from the floor and walk your legs in toward your torso until your torso is perpendicular to the floor. Press into your forearms as you bend both knees into the chest, then extend the feet up toward the ceiling, straightening your legs.

Backbends

In yoga, a back-bending pose is any pose that arches the spine backward. Backbends are invigorating. Plus, they open the chest, which is a mood enhancer. Put these two effects together, and you get stress reduction. It's all good.

You don't have to do a full gymnastic-type classic backbend to receive the benefits—nor should you, unless you are a fairly advanced yoga practitioner or have a similar physical practice. Backbends progress in intensity, from just mildly arching the back all through the spectrum to the full gymnastic-type backbends. As with inversions, you can choose any of the backbends that are safe and appropriate for your level of practice to gain the stress-reduction benefit.

Setu Bandha Sarvangasana, or **Bridge Pose**, is a moderate backbend that can be safely practiced by most beginners. It is one of the most therapeutic yoga poses, and it gives the invigorating effect of back bending while opening the chest. It also strengthens the lower back and relieves tightness in the neck and upper back. As I mentioned before, I like its efficiency—it can serve as a counterpose to Headstand if you are pressed for time.

SETU BANDHA SARVANGASANA (BRIDGE POSE): Recline on your back with your arms along your sides, palms down. Bend your knees and bring your feet hip-width apart, with your heels close to your buttocks. Press down into your feet as you lift your buttocks up toward the ceiling, bringing your chest toward your chin. Roll your shoulders under you and clasp your hands.

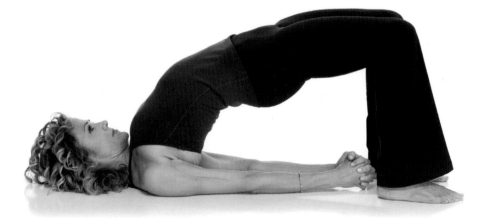

Urdhva Mukha Svanasana, or **Upward-Facing Dog**, is a moderate backbend appropriate for most beginners. I really like Upward-Facing Dog; not only is it a backbend, but it also strengthens the arms, firms the buttocks, and stretches the abdomen very nicely.

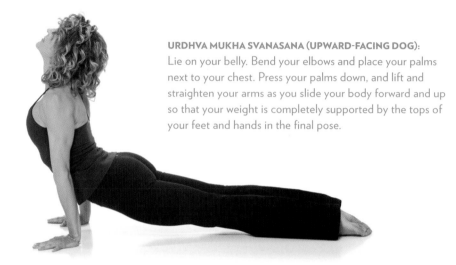

URDHVA MUKHA SVANASANA (UPWARD-FACING DOG):
Lie on your belly. Bend your elbows and place your palms next to your chest. Press your palms down, and lift and straighten your arms as you slide your body forward and up so that your weight is completely supported by the tops of your feet and hands in the final pose.

Bhujangasana, or **Cobra**, is a more advanced backbend than Upward-Facing Dog if it is done correctly (which it frequently is not). That's because Cobra requires you to isolate and use only your back muscles to perform the backbend, whereas in Upward-Facing Dog you have the assistance of your arms and legs. The key to doing Cobra properly is to use your spinal muscles to spiral your torso up into the backbend, using your hands and arms only to stabilize and balance. Cobra strengthens the back and buttocks, and it starts to bring flexibility to the spine.

BHUJANGASANA (COBRA): Lie on your belly. Bend your elbows and place your palms next to your chest. Extend your legs behind you as you use your back muscles to lift your torso up. Press lightly into your palms, using them only to stabilize you in the pose.

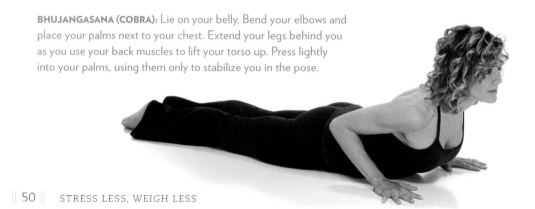

Ustrasana, or **Camel Pose**, is not only a backbend, but a very strong chest opener. It is particularly good for those who work on a computer or drive a lot, because it counterbalances the tightness that generally occurs in the chest muscles from these repetitive activities.

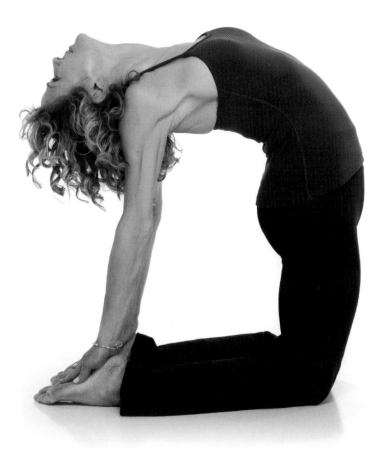

USTRASANA (CAMEL POSE): Kneel on the floor with your knees hip-width apart and your feet pointing dirtectly behind you, with the tops of your feet on the floor. Place your palms on your lower back. Lift your torso as you arch back, then reach your hands to your heels. Draw your hips forward so they are directly over your knees and your thighs are perpendicular to the floor.

Urdhva Dhanurasana, or Upward-Facing Bow Pose, is a full backbend and should be practiced only by more-advanced practitioners. I love this pose. It is a vigorous stretch of the chest and abdomen that strengthens the legs and buttocks, and it is the most invigorating of the backbends.

Backbends never fail to energize me. And a note of caution: I rarely do them later in the evening because of this. I want my sleep!

URDHVA DHANURASANA (UPWARD-FACING BOW): Lie on your back, bend your knees, and bring your heels close to your buttocks. Bend your elbows overhead and place your palms on the floor next to your head, with your fingers pointing toward your feet. Press firmly down into your feet and hands, and lift your hips and chest up toward the ceiling. Straighten your arms and stretch your legs.

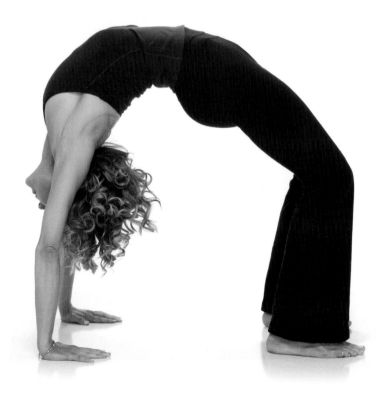

Twists

Twists are excellent to do after backbends because they neutralize the spine, meaning they provide relief. They restore the spine's natural range of motion, stretch the back muscles, and work the abdominal muscles. I don't know if it has been medically proven that twists wring out excess emotion, but I do know that they calm my nerves, leaving me with a soothing tranquillity. Plus, they're easy to do anywhere. You can even do them in your office chair.

Choose any twist that appeals to you and is appropriate for your level of practice. **Jathara Parivartanasana Variation**, or **Reclined Twist**, is a relaxing twist that most beginners can safely practice. It stretches the spine, opens the shoulders and hips, and relieves tension in the lower back. Because you lie down on your back to do it, you can hold it for longer periods than the other twists, which provides more benefit.

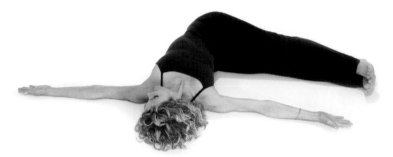

JATHARA PARIVARTANASANA (RECLINED TWIST): Lie on your back with your arms extended, palms up. Bring your knees to your chest, then straighten your legs so they are perpendicular to the floor. Lower your legs to the right, either allowing them to rest on the floor or holding them a few inches from the floor. Hold for twenty to thirty seconds. Repeat on the left.

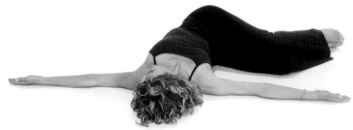

JATHARA PARIVARTANASANA VARIATION (RECLINED TWIST VARIATION): Lie on your back with your knees bent and feet on the floor. Extend your arms straight out from your shoulders in a T position, palms up. Draw your knees to your chest, then roll your knees across your body to the right, bringing your legs to rest on the floor. Hold for at least thirty seconds, then repeat on the left.

Bharadvajasana is a simple seated twist that most beginners can safely practice also. It stretches the spine, shoulders, and hips, and can help relieve back pain.

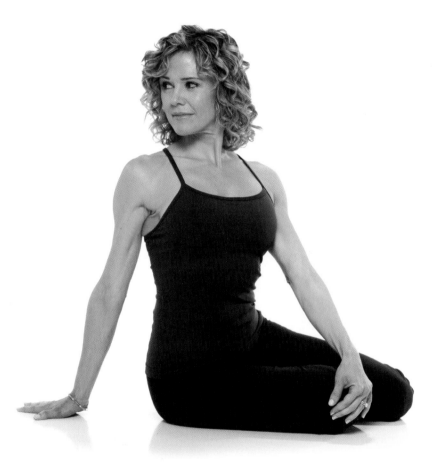

BHARADVAJASANA (SIMPLE SEATED TWIST): Sit with your legs extended in front of you. Bend your knees, draw your feet to the left near your left hip, and release your knees to the floor so they point in front of you. Bring your left hand to your right knee, and reach your right hand to the floor behind you. Inhale and extend up through your torso; exhale and twist to the right. Hold for at least thirty seconds, then repeat on the other side.

Marichyasana III is a slightly more advanced seated twist and one that you've likely seen in group exercise classes at the gym. It too stretches the spine, shoulders, and hips, and it can also help relieve back pain.

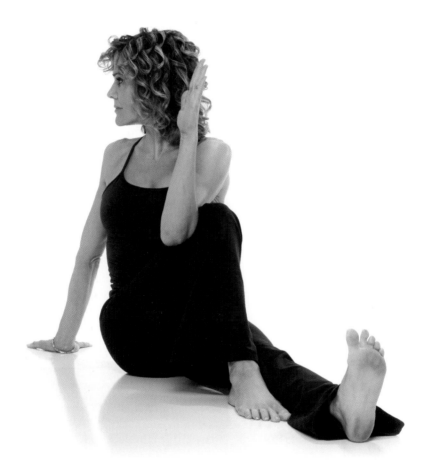

MARICHYASANA III (SEATED TWIST): Sit with your legs extended in front of you. Bend your right knee and bring your right foot to the floor close to your right buttock. Reach your right arm behind you, and place your right hand on the floor. Inhale and extend your left arm straight up. As you exhale, twist to the right and bend your left arm, hooking your left elbow on the outside of your right knee. Hold for thirty seconds, then repeat on the other side.

Ardha Matsyendrasana, or Half Lord of the Fish Pose, is a more advanced twist. It stretches the shoulders, neck, and back, and it gives a greater stretch to the hips than the previous twists. This twist is also more invigorating than the previous twists.

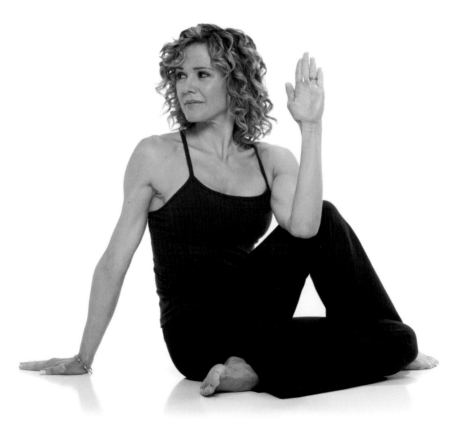

ARDHA MATSYENDRASANA (HALF LORD OF THE FISH POSE): Sit in a kneeling position on the floor with your knees together. Shift your weight to the left, bringing your left buttock to the floor. Leave the left leg where it is as you bend the right leg and cross your right foot over your left leg, bringing your right foot to the floor on the outside of your left thigh. The right knee is pointing up toward the ceiling. Inhale and extend your left arm. Exhale and twist to the right, bending your left elbow and hooking it on the outside of your right thigh and reaching your right hand to the floor behind you. Hold for twenty to thirty seconds, then repeat on the other side.

Baddha Ardha Matsyendrasana, or Bound Half Lord of the Fish Pose, is the most advanced seated twist. It maximizes the stretch to the shoulders, neck, back, and hips. It can take years to be able to get into this pose, but it is well worth the effort. It is my favorite seated twist.

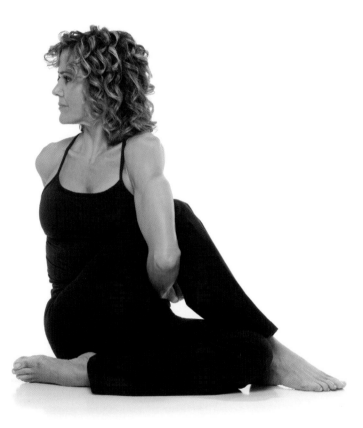

BADDHA ARDHA MATSYENDRASANA (BOUND HALF LORD OF THE FISH POSE): Sit in a kneeling position on the floor with your knees together. Shift your weight to the left, bringing your left buttock to the floor. Leave the left leg where it is as you bend the right leg and cross your right foot over your left leg, bringing your right foot to the floor on the outside of your left thigh. The right knee is pointing up toward the ceiling. Inhale and extend your left arm. Exhale and twist to the right, threading your left arm and hand through your bent right leg as you reach your right arm behind you. Grasp your right hand (or wrist) with your left hand. Now you are in the bind. Hold for twenty to thirty seconds, then repeat on the other side.

Closing pose: Savasana (Corpse Pose)

Savasana, or **Corpse Pose**, applies to all levels. It is the last pose for every yoga sequence, whether beginner, intermediate, or advanced. Savasana, sometimes referred to as Final Relaxation, is a complete stilling of the body and mind, allowing our bodies to assimilate the benefits of the yoga sequence.

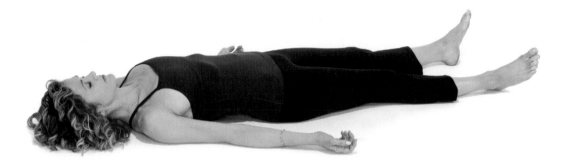

SAVASANA (CORPSE POSE): Lie on your back. Extend your legs and allow your feet to roll out to a comfortable position. Extend your arms next to your body (but not touching your body) with your palms up and fingers relaxed. Close your eyes and breathe naturally. Completely release any muscular tension. Allow your face to be soft, with your jaw slightly parted. Remain here for at least a few minutes, or as long as you like. To come out of the pose, bend your knees to your chest, then roll to your right side, coming into a fetal position for a few breaths. Then, using your palms, press into the floor and come up into a comfortable seated position.

Remember, you can string together any of the above poses to create your own ten-minute sequence, or you can follow my suggested Ten-Minute Beginner Yoga Sequence, Intermediate Yoga Sequence, or Advanced Yoga Sequence (which I give you next). You should hold each pose for at least five long breaths, and for some, much longer. For the longer holds, I'll prompt you in the sequences.

TEN-MINUTE **BEGINNER** YOGA SEQUENCE

Begin in **Tadasana (Mountain Pose)**. Bring your big toes together, heels slightly apart. Lift through the crown of your head as you reach your hands toward the floor. Take a few deep breaths, inhaling and exhaling evenly through the nose.

Next, come to your hands and knees on the mat, with your hands directly under your shoulders and knees hip-width apart. On an exhale, sink your hips to your heels, and reach out with the arms, coming into **Utthita Balasana (Extended Child's Pose)**. Hold for five long breaths. Inhale, and reach the buttocks up and back, and straighten the legs, coming into **Adho Mukha Svanasana (Downward-Facing Dog Pose)**. Hold for five breaths. Exhale, and bring the knees back to the floor, sink the hips to the heels, coming back into **Utthita Balasana (Extended Child's Pose)**. Repeat this sequence five times, moving from **Utthita Balasana** to **Adho Mukha Svanasana**.

Next, lie flat on your stomach with your legs together and toes pointed behind you. Bend your elbows, placing your palms flat on the floor next to your ribs. Press down through your palms, raising your head and chest into **Bhujangasana (Cobra Pose)**. Remain here for five breaths, then lower to the mat to rest. Repeat two more times.

Lie flat on your stomach. We are going to move into **Urdhva Mukha Svanasana (Upward-Facing Dog Pose)**. Just as in **Bhujangasana (Cobra Pose)**, bend your elbows, placing your palms flat on the floor next to your ribs. Press down through your palms and the tops of your feet, drawing your chest forward as you straighten your arms and lift your head, chest, torso, and legs off the ground. Hold for five breaths. Repeat two times.

Next, lie flat on your back, face up. It's time to do our twists, the bent-knee variation of **Jathara Parivartanasana (Reclined Twist)**. Bring the arms out to each side at shoulder level, in a T position, palms up. Draw the knees to the chest, keeping your back on the mat. On an exhale, gently roll your knees to your right side, allowing them to rest on the floor. Take five long, deep breaths. Repeat to the left.

We'll finish by coming into **Savasana (Corpse Pose)**. Lie on your back, extend your legs, and allow your feet to roll open. Extend your arms near your body, with your palms up. Close your eyes and breathe naturally. Completely let go, releasing any muscular tension. You can remain in **Savasana** as long as you like.

TEN-MINUTE **BEGINNER** YOGA SEQUENCE

1. Tadasana (Mountain Pose)

2. Utthita Balasana (Extended Child's Pose)

3. Adho Mukha Svanasana
   (Downward-Facing Dog Pose)

4. Utthita Balasana (Extended Child's Pose)

Repeat steps 3–4 five times, moving from
Utthita Balasana to Adho Mukha Svanasana.

5. Bhujangasana (Cobra Pose)

6. Urdhva Mukha Svanasana
   (Upward-Facing Dog Pose)

7. Jathara Parivartanasana
   (Reclined Twist Variation)

8. Savasana (Corpse Pose)

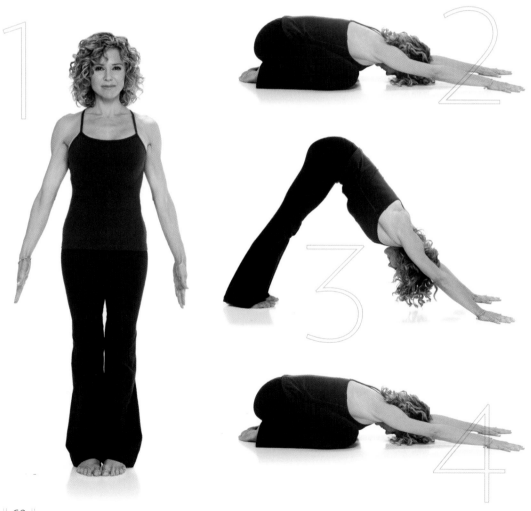

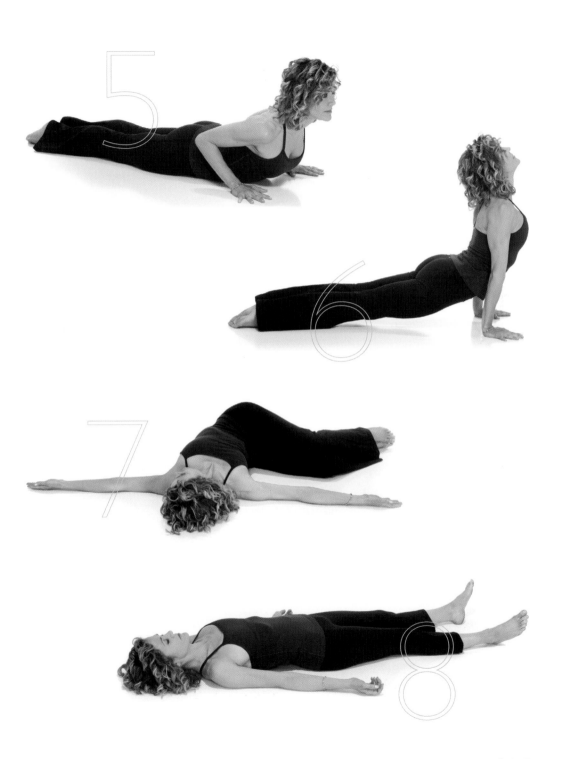

TEN-MINUTE **INTERMEDIATE** YOGA SEQUENCE

Begin in **Tadasana (Mountain Pose)**. Bring your big toes together, heels slightly apart. Lift through the crown of your head as you reach your hands toward the floor. Take a few deep breaths here, inhaling and exhaling evenly through the nose.

Inhale and lift your arms straight up, pause, and reach for the ceiling. Exhale and bring your arms down, coming back into **Tadasana (Mountain Pose)**. Inhale to lift your arms up again, pausing as you really reach for the ceiling. Exhale to come back to **Tadasana**. Repeat this sequence three more times.

Place your mat perpendicular to a wall. Kneel down, with your head toward the wall, and come to your hands and knees on the mat, with your hands directly under your shoulders, and knees hip-width apart. Your hands should be about six inches away from the wall.

On an inhale, reach the buttocks up and back, and straighten the legs, coming into **Adho Mukha Svanasana (Downward-Facing Dog Pose)**. Hold for five breaths. Walk your feet forward until your shoulders are perpendicular to your wrists. Bend one leg under your chest in a lunge position, and raise the other leg to prepare to kick up. Kick up with the bent leg as you swing the raised leg up. Reach both heels to the wall, coming into **Adho Mukha Vrksasana (Handstand)**. Try to hold Handstand as long as you can, aiming for at least five deep breaths.

On an exhale, bring your legs down, and come back into **Adho Mukha Svanasana (Downward-Facing Dog Pose)**. Hold for five breaths, then walk forward again to go back into **Adho Mukha Vrksasana (Handstand)**. Again, try to hold Handstand as long as you can.

Repeat the sequence from **Adho Mukha Svansana (Downward-Facing Dog Pose)** to **Adho Mukha Vrksasana (Handstand)** and back to **Adho Mukha Svansana (Downward-Facing Dog Pose)** one more time.

From **Adho Mukha Svansana (Downward-Facing Dog Pose)**, exhale, bring the knees back to the floor, sink the hips to the heels, and reach out with your arms, coming into **Utthita Balasana (Extended Child's Pose)**. Take a few breaths here to rest.

It is now time to do our backbends. We're going to do three rounds of **Ustrasana (Camel Pose)**. Kneel on the floor with your knees hip-width apart and your feet

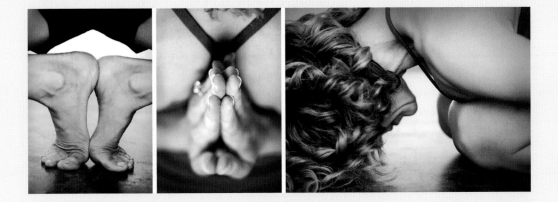

pointing directly behind you, with the tops of your feet on the floor. Place your palms on your lower back. Lift your torso as you arch back, then reach your hands to your heels. Draw your hips forward so they are directly over your knees and your thighs are perpendicular to the floor. Hold for five breaths. Come out of the pose by walking your hands up to your hips. Take a few recovery breaths, then repeat **Ustrasana** once or twice.

For our closing twists, we will do **Ardha Matsyendrasana (Half Lord of the Fish Pose)**. Sit in a kneeling position on the floor with your knees together. Shift your weight to the left, bringing your left buttock to the floor. Leave the left leg where it is as you bend the right leg and cross your right foot over your left leg, bringing your right foot to the floor on the outside of your left thigh. The right knee is pointing up toward the ceiling. Inhale and extend your left arm. Exhale and twist to the right, bending your left elbow and hooking it on the outside of your right thigh and reaching your right hand to the floor behind you. Hold for twenty to thirty seconds, then repeat on the other side.

We're going to finish the sequence by coming into **Savasana (Corpse Pose)**. Lie on your back, extend your legs, and allow your feet to roll open. Extend your arms near your body, with your palms up. Close your eyes and breathe naturally. Completely let go and unwind, releasing any muscular tension. You can remain in **Savasana** as long as you like.

TEN-MINUTE INTERMEDIATE YOGA SEQUENCE

1. Tadasana (Mountain Pose)
2. Adho Mukha Svanasana
   (Downward-Facing Dog Pose)
3. Adho Mukha Vrksasana (Handstand)

Repeat steps 2–3 two times, moving from Adho Mukha Svanasana to Adho Mukha Vrksasana.

4. Utthita Balasana (Extended Child's Pose)
5. Ustrasana (Camel Pose)

Repeat Ustrasana one or two times.

6. Ardha Matsyendrasana
   (Half Lord of the Fish Pose)
7. Savasana (Corpse Pose)

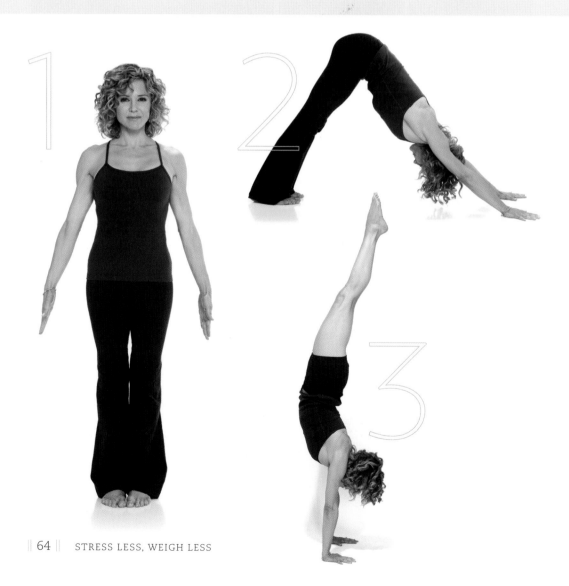

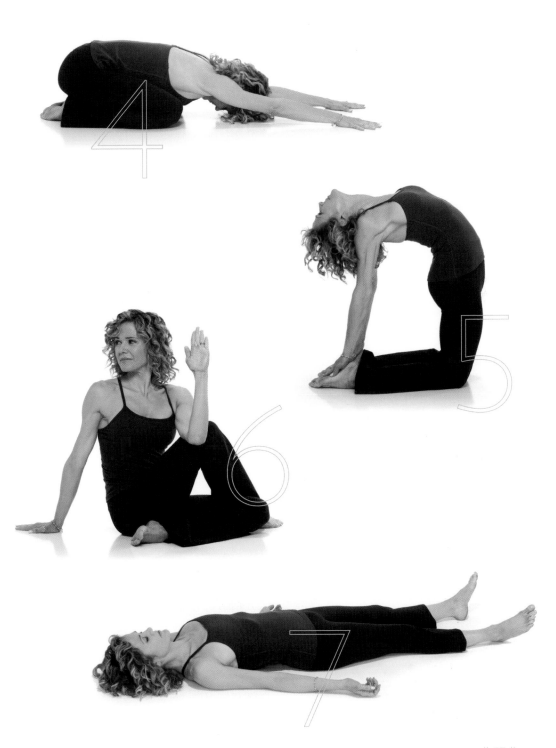

TEN-MINUTE **ADVANCED** YOGA SEQUENCE

Begin in **Tadasana (Mountain Pose)**. Bring your big toes together, heels slightly apart. Lift through the crown of your head as you reach your hands toward the floor. Take a few deep breaths, inhaling and exhaling evenly through the nose.

Inhale and lift your arms straight up, pause, and reach for the ceiling. Exhale and bring your arms down, coming back into **Tadasana (Mountain Pose)**. Inhale to lift your arms up again, pausing as you really reach for the ceiling. Exhale to come back to **Tadasana**. Repeat this sequence three more times.

We are going to go into **Sirsasana (Headstand)**. Place your mat perpendicular to a wall. Come to your hands and knees. Bend your arms and bring your elbows to the floor, shoulder-width apart. Interlace your fingers and cup your hands. Your hands should be at, or very near, the baseboard. Place the crown of your head on the floor with your hands lightly cupping the back of your head. Lift your knees from the floor and walk your legs in toward your torso until your torso is perpendicular to the floor. Press into your forearms as you bend both knees into the chest, then extend the feet up toward the ceiling, straightening your legs.

Try to hold **Sirsasana Headstand** at least one minute, and better yet, longer if you can. It is a tremendous strength builder and stress reducer.

When you are ready to come down, firm your core and slowly bring both feet to the floor. Leaving your head on the mat, come directly into **Utthita Balasana (Extended Child's Pose)** by sinking your hips to your heels, bringing your forehead to the floor, and reaching out with your arms. Rest here for at least five to ten long breaths.

Now that our inversions are complete, we will move on to backbends. But it is important to counterbalance a headstand. The perfect pose to meet both needs is **Setu Bandha Sarvangasana (Bridge Pose)** because it provides a nice stretch to the back of the neck as well as being a mild backbend.

To come into **Setu Bandha Sarvangasana (Bridge Pose)**, recline on your back with your arms along your sides, palms down. Bend your knees and bring your feet hip-width apart, with your heels close to your buttocks. Press down into your feet as you lift your buttocks up toward the ceiling, bringing your chest toward your chin. Roll your shoulders under you and clasp your hands. Hold for five long breaths. Release your hands and slowly lower your body down, rest for a few breaths, then repeat.

Our final backbend is **Urdhva Dhanurasana (Upward-Facing Bow Pose)**. Lie on your back, bend your knees, and bring your heels close to your buttocks. Bend your elbows overhead and place your palms on the floor next to your head, with your fingers pointing toward your feet. Press firmly down into your feet and hands, and lift your hips and chest up toward the ceiling. Straighten your arms and stretch your legs. Hold the pose for five deep breaths. Come down, take a few recovery breaths, then repeat the pose.

After your final **Urdhva Dhanurasana (Upward-Facing Bow Pose)**, remain lying on your back, draw your knees to your chest, and slowly rock from side to side to relieve your back.

We'll finish with an advanced twist, **Baddha Ardha Matsyendrasana (Bound Half Lord of the Fish Pose)**. Sit in a kneeling position on the floor with your knees together. Shift your weight to the left, bringing your left buttock to the floor. Leave the left leg where it is as you bend the right leg and cross your right foot over your left leg, bringing your right foot to the floor on the outside of your left thigh. The right knee is pointing up toward the ceiling. Inhale and extend your left arm. Exhale and twist to the right, threading your left arm and hand through your bent right leg, as you reach your right arm behind you. Grasp your right hand (or wrist) with your left hand. Now you are in the bind. Hold for twenty to thirty seconds, then repeat on the other side.

The final pose is **Savasana (Corpse Pose)**, so we can absorb and integrate the effects of this vigorous sequence. Lie on your back, extend your legs, and allow your feet to roll open. Extend your arms near your body, with your palms up. Close your eyes and breathe naturally. Completely let go and unwind, releasing any muscular tension. You can remain in **Savasana** as long as you like.

TEN-MINUTE ADVANCED YOGA SEQUENCE

1. Tadasana (Mountain Pose)

2. Sirsasana (Headstand)

3. Utthita Balasana (Extended Child's Pose)

4. Setu Bandha Sarvangasana (Bridge Pose)

5. Urdhva Dhanurasana
   (Upward-Facing Bow Pose)

Repeat Urdhva Dhanurasana once.

6. Baddha Ardha Matsyendrasana
   (Bound Half Lord of the Fish Pose)

7. Savasana (Corpse Pose)

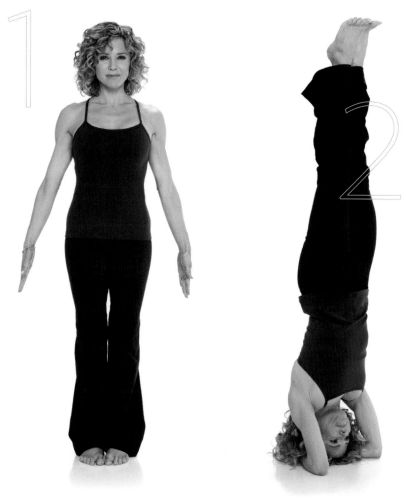

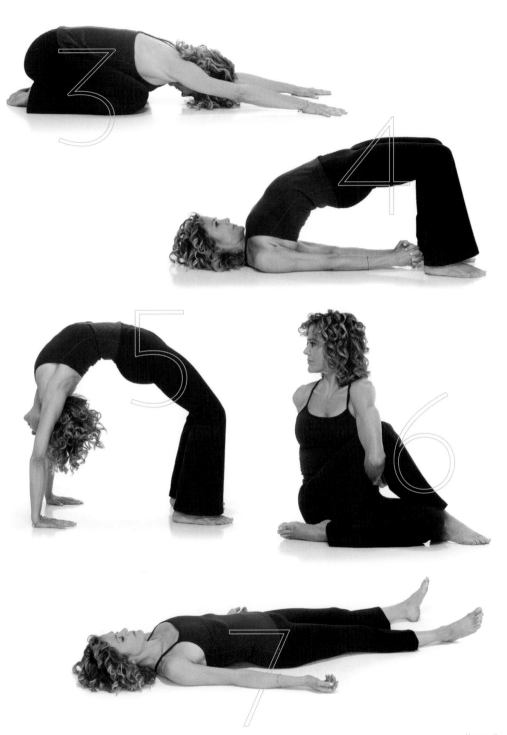

RESTORATIVE YOGA—
A STRESS-RELIEVER IN A CLASS OF ITS OWN

Restorative yoga is designed to do just that—restore you. It is a premier stress reducer, and it replenishes mind, body, and soul. However, I have found that ten minutes of restorative yoga is not sufficient to get the real benefits it can bestow. I need at least thirty minutes of it (and more if I have time) to experience the restorative effects. I'll give you my go-to Thirty-Minute Restorative Yoga Sequence on the following pages.

In restorative yoga the poses are passive, meaning you are not using muscle and balance to hold them. Generally, you are in a reclined position using props such as bolsters, pillows, and blankets to support you in the pose. You are not exerting energy for this practice. Instead, you receive energy. The focus is on long holds (around three to five minutes each) so you can fully receive the benefits the poses have to offer.

Make no mistake—although the poses look (and are) very mild, the results are anything but. Holding these mild backbends, twists, and forward folds for the recommended three to five minutes each is not hard at all, but the intense relaxation available from a restorative practice sinks deep into the nervous system, enhancing blood circulation, releasing chronic muscle tension, and triggering the parasympathetic nervous system to the relaxation response.

Rather than wait until I actually "need" a restorative yoga session, I like to be proactive and try to do one of these sessions every week (or at least every other week) as one of my regular stress-management tools. Why wait until I am depleted? When you experience how good these restorative poses feel, you'll see that although they appear very mild, they afford a distinct and immediate soothing effect. A restorative session is a major tool for building a reserve of calm to draw from in more stressful times.

I have also found restorative yoga to be extremely helpful when I am traveling. I like to do a thirty-minute session the day I arrive in my hotel to settle in. Because these poses invoke the relaxation response, they are ideal to do before bed, if that's when you get to them.

And a restorative practice is always recommended for women on their menstrual cycles, particularly on the first day of the cycle. It is also a perfect practice to do if you are recovering from an illness or injury. But again, and this goes for everyone—men and women—a once-a-week restorative yoga session will ward off all manner of ills and aggravation, and it's an easy and enjoyable proactive stress-management tool.

MY THIRTY-MINUTE RESTORATIVE YOGA SEQUENCE

I always combine pranayama (focused breathing) with my restorative practice. It amplifies the relaxation effect. So in the sequence that follows, I will prompt you on the breath. I do a simple pranayama—the same one I told you about in Chapter Two, the Four-Count Breath—then after a bit I add in the breath retention as I taught you in that section.

Let's begin.

We'll start in **Supported Savasana (Supported Corpse Pose).** Recline on your mat. Place two narrowly folded blankets (or one, if you prefer) under your knees and another folded blanket under your head. (Try using beach towels if you don't have blankets.)

Close your eyes, and let your breath be normal. Take a few minutes to slowly scan your body from your toes to the crown of your head, releasing any tension you find. Once you are completely still and relaxed, spend another minute or two here, allowing your body to sink into your mat.

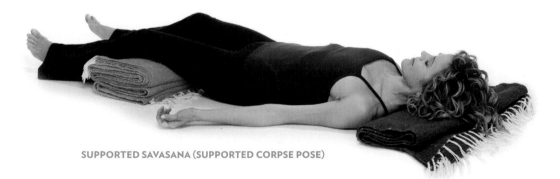

SUPPORTED SAVASANA (SUPPORTED CORPSE POSE)

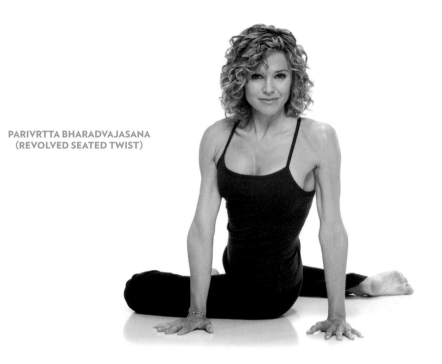

PARIVRTTA BHARADVAJASANA
(REVOLVED SEATED TWIST)

Next, we'll come into a **Parivrtta Bharadvajasana (Revolved Seated Twist)**. Sit up with your knees bent and your feet on the mat, with your feet placed wider than your hips. Let your knees roll to the right as you twist completely to your right side, all the way toward the wall behind you, with your hands on the mat, supporting you. When you fully come into this twist, you will be facing the wall behind you. Begin the Four-Count Breath, and hold the pose for at least five breaths. Slowly release, and repeat on the left side. After that, repeat again on the right side, then the left.

Next, we'll move into **Supported Supta Baddha Konasana (Reclined Bound Angle Pose)**. Stack two narrowly folded blankets. (Fold the blankets the same way we did for Supported Savasana, or Supported Corpse Pose.) Place them vertically on your mat so when you lie back they support your spine. Take another folded blanket and place it horizontally at the top of the vertical blankets. This blanket will be supporting your head. Sit on your mat, and place your lower back against the vertical blankets. Draw the soles of your feet together and let your knees fall open (if you have a tight groin or this is uncomfortable, you can place folded blankets or pillows under each knee for support). Slowly recline back, resting the center of your spine in the middle of the vertical blankets and resting your head on the horizontal blanket.

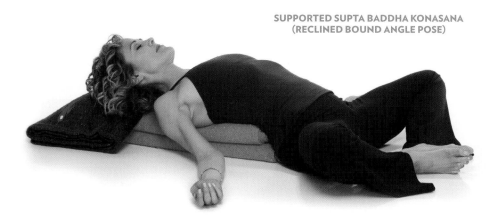

SUPPORTED SUPTA BADDHA KONASANA
(RECLINED BOUND ANGLE POSE)

Bring your arms out to the side to open your chest. Close your eyes.

You're going to remain here for five minutes. As soon as you settle in, begin the Four-Count Breath, breathing in through your nose to the count of four, then exhaling through your nose to the count of four. After several of these breaths, begin to extend the breath to the count of five or six, making the count of your inhale match the count of your exhale.

Take your time. Once you are comfortable extending the breath to the count of five or six, add breath retention. Breathe in and retain the breath in for a count of two, then exhale and retain the breath out for a count of two. Do this for at least another five to ten breaths (or more), unless you feel a strain. If it is a strain to do the breath retention, skip it.

After at least five of these breaths, go back to normal breathing.

To come out of the pose, use your hands to bring your knees together. Roll off the blankets to your right side, and remain here in a fetal position for a few breaths. Then using your hands, slowly press yourself up.

Now we are going to do a **Supported Side Twist**. Fold three or four blankets in quarters. Sit on your mat, with your legs straight in front of you. Stack the blankets horizontally, next to your right hip. Bend your left leg back. Place your hands on either side of your blankets, and twist to the right so your torso is centered over the blankets. Slowly lower your torso to the blankets and turn your face to one side, resting your cheek on the blankets and letting the blankets fully support you.

Wiggle around a bit until you find a comfortable position so you can fully relax in the pose. This is a fairly intense twist, so take your time to find your way into it. You will be here for five minutes.

Once you are comfortable, begin the Four-Count Breath, breathing in through your nose to the count of four, then exhaling through your nose to the count of four. You may notice it is a bit more difficult to breathe deeply while in this twist because your diaphragm is not fully free to easily expand. That's okay—just stick with it, but don't strain. You are gaining an additional benefit by the breath affecting, and massaging, your internal organs in a slightly different position. In yoga, twisting postures are believed to massage the internal organs, bringing enhanced circulation and vitality to them, and to restore flexibility to the spine. I believe that adding the pranayama to these twists boosts those effects.

If you can get comfortable with the Four-Count Breath, go ahead and try extending the inhales and exhales to the count of five or six, as we did with the other poses. Once you are comfortable with extending the breath, add a count or two of breath retention, retaining the breath in for one or two counts after you inhale, then retaining the breath out for one or two counts after you exhale. After a few of these, go back to breathing normally and comfortably.

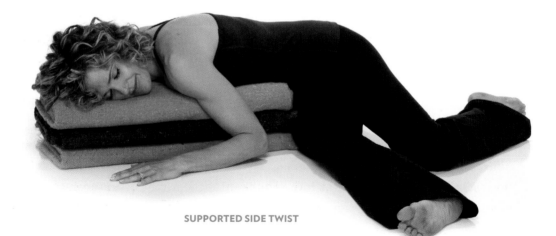

SUPPORTED SIDE TWIST

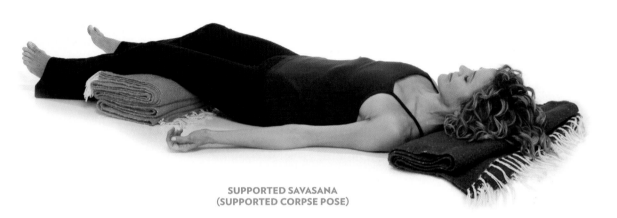

**SUPPORTED SAVASANA
(SUPPORTED CORPSE POSE)**

Now switch sides and perform the twist on your left side. Hold the twist for five minutes and do the same pranayama on the left side as you did on the right side.

We'll end the way we started—in **Supported Savasana (Supported Corpse Pose)**. Recline on your mat with the folded blankets under your knees and another blanket under your head. Close your eyes and let your breath be normal. Take a few minutes to slowly scan your body from your toes to the crown of your head, releasing any tension you find. Once you are completely still and relaxed, spend a final minute or two here, allowing your body to sink into your mat. Give yourself time—at least five minutes; you want to allow your body to fully absorb and integrate the benefits of this restorative practice.

To finish, roll to your right side and remain in a fetal position for a few breaths. Then use your hands to press yourself up to a comfortable seated position. Keep your eyes closed, and reestablish the Four-Count Breath for several breaths. Then slowly open your eyes. Before you move, form an internal intent to take the calming effects of this practice with you into the rest of your day.

WHAT IF I DON'T LIKE
ANYTHING I'VE SEEN HERE?

Don't worry if you haven't seen something here that interests you. Yoga offers something for everyone. When I first began taking yoga teacher training, a dear friend of mine (who once said she hated yoga) timidly asked me if I was going to stop shaving my armpits and start wearing Birkenstocks.

This is a common misperception held by people who are unfamiliar with the multitude of yoga styles and the great variety of people who teach and practice it. Sure, you can find earthier teachers and groups if you are drawn to that. I've been to the classes where the women don't shave their armpits. But I personally enjoy a more vigorous "flow" type of yoga practice that many people from the corporate world are drawn to.

I also like to mix in regular Iyengar classes to keep the integrity in my alignment, because I have found that when I take only flow-type classes, I tend to get a little sloppy. In the Iyengar classes, there's a different philosophy, different instruction, and there tends to be a whole different group of students. I still intend to explore Yin yoga, Kunda-lini yoga, and take some more Viniyoga and Anusara classes . . . The list goes on and on. Again, there's something for everyone.

That's why I encourage you to seek a yoga practice that appeals to you and fits comfortably into your lifestyle. Chances are, there's one that's right for you. If you are like me, the Ten-Minute Yoga Sequences may end up forming the foundation of your yoga practice. And that is perfectly okay.

But even if you opt for a different path altogether, be sure you find something that helps you counteract stress and build a cushion of peace in your schedule.

I have observed that whenever there is a lack of space, whether in the body, mind, or life path, there is debilitation of the surrounding structure. A mind that is thinking incessantly breaks down in its ability to think clearly. A body with no space for stillness and rest shows evidence of the ravages of time much sooner and to a greater degree than one that walks through life embraced in a buffer of space.

When it comes to how much space we give ourselves, perhaps most telling is the

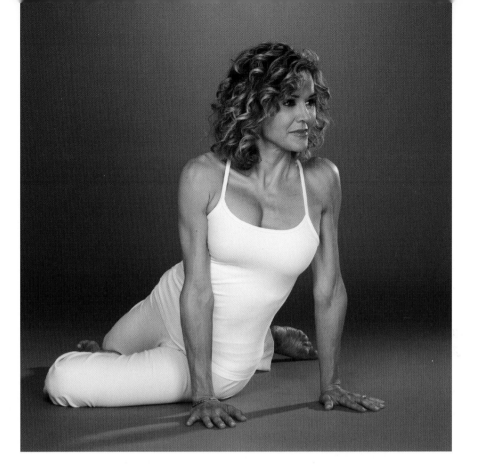

evidence that our careers and family life provide. Without time for contemplation and introspection, our trail is only a collection of knee-jerk reactions to events and circumstances, because there has been no reflection that would allow us to choose a more fulfilling and meaningful path.

I like yoga for this reason. Yes, it definitely reduces stress. I think it does this by bringing space into my body. Muscle tightness and tension dissipate as I extend and reach, opening my shoulders, neck, and hips. The contracted, taut areas of my body find freedom and boy, does it feel good. I have found I can work from the outside in: When I bring space into my body, I always gain some space in my mind. My thoughts slow. That allows me to move away from old, habitual patterns of thought and reaction. Over time, I find I've created a new life free from the taint of decades of tightly wound automatic responses that clouded my ability to access the wisdom available from the seat of my soul.

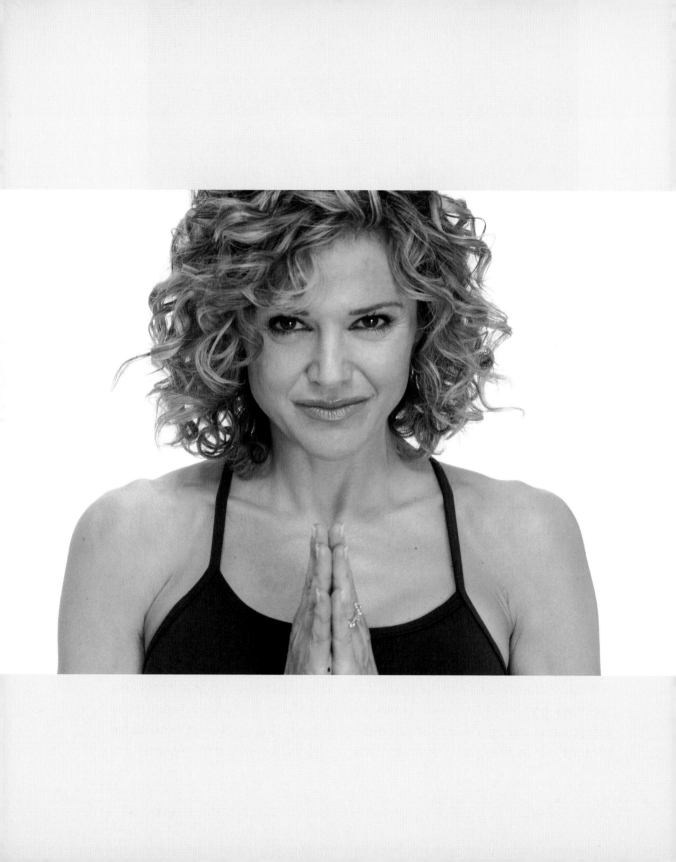

CHAPTER 4

USE MENTAL FOCUS TO ELEVATE YOUR MOOD

What a freeing revelation it was to discover that I was a victim of my own emotions. I saw that all the unrelenting stress and angst I was suffering was caused by my negative thought habits. At that time, I was so dejected that even if something good happened, my mind still turned to what was wrong with it and all my focus went there. Husband cleaned the kitchen before I arrived home? Wonderful, right? But I am ashamed to admit that, I would see only the cookie crumbs on the counter that he forgot to wipe.

Focusing on problems generated negative emotions, and away I went on a downward spiral until all joy had been sucked out of my life—by my own hand. Go figure.

But armed with the awareness that I had led myself to this black hole, I could see that the power to get out was also in my hands. It was up to me to choose to guide my thoughts toward the positives. No one could do it for me. I wasn't the victim of anyone or anything else; until that moment of awareness, I was my own worst enemy, feeding my mind a steady diet of poison and then feeling perplexed as to why I was so overwrought.

Despite my awareness, the way out was not clearly paved. I had to really hunt to find some simple techniques to direct my mental focus toward positive thoughts. But once I did, it was like finding a lantern that illuminated the pathway out. All I had to do was follow the light. Anytime I found myself starting to sink back toward negativity, I just had to make that first effort to use one of my techniques, and the downward spiral was reversed.

Let me walk you through them so you can claim your happiness too.

SWITCH YOUR **FOCUS**

Every time I'm ticked off and stressed out, I know it's because I am focusing on the one or two things that are going wrong instead of the thousands of things that are actually going well. Maybe I had an argument with my husband or an unexpected bill came in. All my focus goes there! But in truth, so many more things are going right. I still have my health, my family, my car, food in my refrigerator. I have my house, a warm bed to sleep in at night. You get the picture. We allow our thoughts to dwell on the couple of negatives, giving them much more weight than they deserve, and we just dismiss the overwhelming positives. Think about it. Isn't that true for you too? So this is another very effective stress tool: Switch Your Focus. Turn your attention to all of the things that are going right in your life. Like attracts like. Once you start focusing on the positive, you'll start noticing more positive thoughts and feelings. We just need to take that first step.

Try it for yourself. Take any positive thought—anything that makes you feel good or happy, something you feel grateful for—and just ponder it for a moment. See how quickly similar thoughts flood in? On the flip side, be alert when you feel bad. Try to take a bystander position, and notice how one negative thought just follows the next without any effort. And then the next time you feel nasty, intervene. You have the power to switch tracks, moving your train of thought from the negative to the positive. It really is that simple, but it's not easy. We have spent a lifetime allowing our thoughts to run rampant in any direction, forming the long-term habit of being victims of our thoughts rather than mastering them. But this destructive habit of allowing our thoughts to run away with us can—and must—be changed if we are ever to have a consistently peaceful and stress-free life.

Thoughts are like magnets. The positive ones attract more positive ones. The negative ones attract more negative ones. And thoughts, in turn, create our emotions.

WE GENERATE OUR EMOTIONS

Emotions don't just land on us. We generate them. Every emotion we feel was triggered by a thought. Stop here for a moment and check it out for yourself. Do you get happy for no reason, or do you get happy *after* thinking about something that pleases you? What about when you feel miserable? Isn't that triggered by first thinking about something that displeased you? I know this is true for me.

Because I know that my emotions will flow from my thoughts, I focus on improving my thoughts rather than scrambling to apply first aid to my feelings, which, unfortunately, our culture encourages us to do. It's not that I don't think we should employ methods to soothe our feelings; I do. I just think we get way too indulgent with our feelings, endlessly ruminating and wrestling with them, rather than working on the underlying thoughts that generated the unwanted emotions in the first place. I have yet to see how wallowing in emotion benefits us. Have you ever known anyone with no control over his or her feelings who had any semblance of a peaceful life? I certainly haven't. I try to avoid people with uncontrolled emotions. Those are the people I refer to as loose cannons because they exercise no control over what they lob at others, under the guise that they can't control their feelings.

What we most definitely have control over is our thoughts. We do have a choice in what we're going to think about, and how we are going to think about it, even though we may exercise that choice infrequently. Instead, for some reason, we humans like to fall into a victim mentality. It's easier to think, against all evidence to the contrary, that we feel good or bad because of something that's happened. Not true. We choose what to think and how to react to circumstances, and that includes how we feel. Your personal perspective of an event colors your thoughts about it, and those thoughts, in turn, result in the emotions you feel.

And don't even get me started on that old pop psychobabble that "feelings are neither good or bad, they just *are*." What a load of garbage. Feelings, or emotions, that feel bad and cause us to act badly are *bad*. Why entertain them when we can chose better thoughts and massage those attendant emotions into ones that are positive and motivate us to be an uplifting force in our own lives and in the lives of others? I refuse to be a victim of my own emotions, and you should refuse to be a victim of yours too. Life got much, much better for me when I realized that if I made the effort to guide my thoughts to positive things, I had happy feelings. Happy feelings are stress free.

To help me govern my thoughts and guide them away from a negative point of view, it has helped me immensely to realize that, whatever my perspective or opinion on something, it is based on incomplete information. I'm not omniscient. I perceive this world through imperfect sensory organs. Our eyes can perceive only a minute potion of the colors that actually exist. Our ears hear only a narrow range of the ongoing vibrations around us. In the practical sense, I cannot possibly know all of the facts and circumstances that led up to something happening; I know only the limited range of information I personally had access to. And many times, my personal information was derived from other people—who strained the information through their own filter (usually unknowingly) before they shared it with me. So now I have multiple levels of misperception feeding my view of things.

IF YOU ARE GOING TO ASSUME, ASSUME THE BEST

Not only is the information we receive already somewhat warped by imperfect perception, but being human, we also unconsciously infuse a whole lot of assumptions into it. For example, let's say somebody says something we don't like. Instead of just leaving it at that—a statement was made that we don't agree with, and therefore we dismiss it from our minds—we start mentally investigating the reasons why we think that person said it: "I think she said that because she doesn't like me," or "I probably said something that made him mad." Perhaps none of these assumptions are true, and the other person was upset or distracted by something completely unrelated to us. But we make it personal, then ruminate about it, then generate negative emotion, then attract more negative thoughts. And then we're stressed—but we've created that stress ourselves!

What happened here is that we observed a very limited amount of information and assumed the rest. Assumptions are rarely helpful and usually harmful. As the old saying goes, "When you assume, you make an ass out of 'u' and 'me.'" I say if we're going to assume at all, why not assume the best? What's the harm in that? Have you ever been sorry that you mistakenly assumed that although someone said or did something you didn't like, the person had a good intention or good reason for doing it? Whether the individual did or didn't have good intentions doesn't matter; it doesn't hurt me at all to presume they did—it helps me. That thought elevates my mind and generates feel-good emotions. So I'm going there. It's a much less dramatic way to live, that's for sure. And less drama equals less stress.

Moreover, I am aware that the opinions and assumptions I hold color everything I perceive, slotting the new information into my old mental organizational scheme. I learned this when I was a trial lawyer. No two eyewitnesses perceived the same accident the same way, even if they were standing next to each other. They focused on, and saw, different aspects. We know a juror's past experience colors the opinions that person holds, and the juror will perceive the evidence we present through the filter of preexisting opinions. That's why trial lawyers take so much time questioning potential jurors in voir dire. It's not because we think we will find jurors with no preexisting opinions. That's impossible. We are trying to find the ones who are already slanted, or at least amenable, toward our position.

Put more simply, it's like wearing yellow sunglasses. Everything I see will have a yellow cast to it because I'm looking at it through a colored lens. Even if I'm seeing a new type of blue flower for the first time, it's still going to be tainted by the yellow in my lenses. I would walk away from that experience believing I had just observed my first green flower. And I would be wrong.

This dynamic holds true of everything we perceive. In actuality, there is very little we perceive accurately, yet the human mind is such that it will still form assumptions and opinions that it now insists are the "truth."

This recognition of my imperfect perception has helped me to take myself, my thoughts, and my opinions a heck of a lot less seriously. That helps me have a much lighter attitude and a better mood most of the time, so I am less susceptible to negative thoughts in the first place.

TEST IT FOR YOURSELF

Observe it for yourself and see if it isn't true for you. We don't just decide to feel nasty for no reason. Generally, we feel nasty because we've thought about something unwanted, something negative, that generated an emotion: sadness, anger, fear, or jealousy. I have never found significant relief from emotions unless and until I exercised some discipline over the thoughts that generated them.

Try it. Actively choose what you're going to think about, and I promise you will start improving your mood. You may not think you have the ability in any one moment to "fix" the thing that's bugging you, but who says you have to think about it? Many times, when I switch my focus, I'll forget about what's bugging me. And by the time I revisit the issue, it's resolved.

Years ago Carl Jung, the renowned Swiss psychoanalyst, wrote, "Emotions are contagious." A host of scientific research has since backed that up. Studies have found that the moods of those around us influence our own moods, and vice versa. We infect others with our moods and emotions. So we benefit everyone if we train ourselves to switch our focus to positive things.

IF ALL ELSE FAILS, TRY DISTRACTION

But how do we switch to the positive? Sometimes, in spite of my best intentions, I can't seem to pull out of a negative focus. If I cannot bring myself at that moment to turn my focus to all the things that are going right in my life, I will just find something of an uplifting nature to distract myself away from the negative thought.

Distraction works, but I've learned that a walk still lets me ruminate. Distract yourself with something that requires you to focus. Read a good book or magazine, watch an uplifting program, go to a fun movie. These things help me move toward positive thoughts. So does attending a group exercise class where I have to listen and follow instructions; plus, there's a natural release of endorphins (the feel-good hormones) that comes with exercise. Playing with my dog never fails to cheer me up. Again, research has proven that pets have mood-enhancing and stress-reducing effects on us.

These are some of the methods I use to lift my spirits. Sometimes, once I'm feeling positive again, I'll jot down a list of things that are wonderful in my life and that make me happy. I'll put that list in my purse or pocket and read it over a couple of times until I'm firmly rooted in positive emotions. When I'm happy, I'm not feeling stressed.

So switch your focus. Turn your attention to all of the factors that are going right. The quicker you do this, the more likely you are to avoid that dump of stress hormones into your system, and the attendant cravings for high-fat, high-sugar, and high-sodium foods. And the more you practice this, the more it will become your new conditioned response—a new habit of thought—and you'll feel more positive and less stressed all the time . . .

Which reminds me. Whatever you do to distract yourself from negative thoughts, *stay away from food* during these times. That's an instant binge waiting to happen.

DECIDE HOW YOU ARE GOING TO FEEL ABOUT SOMETHING BEFORE IT HAPPENS

This is an effective stress preventive that has served me extremely well.

I don't know if this is one of those urban legends or not, but the beauty and wisdom of the message is worth passing on. As the story goes, there was an elderly woman whose husband had died, and she was being moved from her lovely family home into a senior citizens' facility. This would be a traumatizing event for most of us.

After she was moved in, she continued with her lifelong habit of getting up early in the morning and grooming herself, then setting about doing whatever her tasks

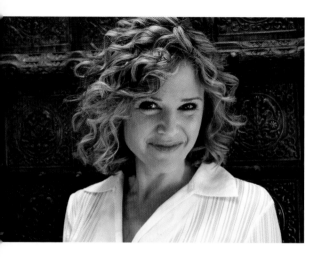

were for that day, whether that was crocheting or writing a letter.

When asked a week after her move how she liked her new "home," she smiled and cheerfully exclaimed, "I love it!" She was then asked how that could be, after losing her husband and home. "My dear," she replied with a smile and twinkle in her eye, "Happiness does not depend on the contents of your surroundings. Happiness depends on the contents of your mind."

She had decided, before her move, that she was going to love it. So that's what she was prepared to do—look for things to love in her new environment. And she found them.

Urban legend or not, I saw my grandmother do the same thing. Grandma Sina was eighty-nine years old when her husband of seventy years died. For more than forty years, she had lived in the family home he built, but it was time to go to an assisted-living facility. Her family packed up the few things that would fit in her new, tiny place, and they distributed the rest of her beloved belongings and heirlooms to family and friends. Then she was shuttled off to her new home.

This could not have been easy for her at all. Many, probably myself included, would have felt fearful and frustrated at having reached such an advanced age, only to lose everything they love.

But not my grandma. True to her lifelong habit of not just making the best of things but deciding how she wanted to feel about something—then working on that, rather than trying to wrestle change out of things that never would—she smoothly sailed through this transition and quickly found the joy she was expecting. Within weeks, she was joining the other ladies for card games and quilting. And she has thrived there for fifteen years, enjoying her life.

The proof? She is 107 years old as I write this—still happy and healthy.

I learned an important lesson from this. We all know you can put two people in the same environment, and one will thrive and find happiness while the other finds endless reasons to complain and be miserable. The difference lies in expectation—and we have control over what we expect.

I recently went to India, a dream of mine for years. I went expecting to love it—and I did. I loved the people, the topography, the food, and the underlying spiritual current I felt coursing through the land. And I kept my focus there during my stay. It wasn't that I didn't see the crushing poverty and horrible sanitary conditions. You can't miss it. (While we were there, the Commonwealth Games were set for the next week in New Delhi. An international uproar had erupted as numerous athletes from other countries exited India before the games because of abysmal sanitary conditions at the athletes' dormitories. A lengthy newspaper article in the national paper, the *Indian Express,* entitled "Brown Terrorism at CWG" discussed in a lively, blunt, and hilarious manner the horrid state of sanitation in India, with the writer declaring that he seeks out five-star hotels to do his "business" and stating that the Indian official in charge of this mess deserved the death penalty.)

So, yes, there was no overlooking this downside of India. We couldn't even walk on the beautiful Arabian Sea beach below our door, so littered with waste it was. But having decided to love India before I arrived, I put my gaze elsewhere. There was so much beauty to see, so much newness for me to absorb and enjoy. I simply lifted my gaze, and my thought, to those things that supported my prior decision. And I had a wonderful time.

So there you have it. With anything coming up on the horizon, *decide before it arrives* how you want feel about it, aiming to view it in the most positive light possible. This does not mean we shouldn't take steps to change or avoid unpleasantries. That we should definitely do, but sometimes that is not an option. Look at my grandma.

I have found this a fabulous stress-prevention tool—proactively moving my head into a calm and peaceful state ahead of the game. I don't wait until I get somewhere or find myself in the middle of something, then react to the input that comes flying at my senses. I mentally prepare beforehand. I *am* open-minded—with a predilection toward expecting and looking for the best the experience has to offer me. It's kind of like the difference between sitting on a buoy in the ocean, bobbing and weaving with every changing wave, or riding a motorboat, speeding toward the course you want your mood to take.

CULTIVATE THE HABIT OF BEING HAPPY

It took me decades to realize that our habitual state of mind is just that—a habit. What an "aha" moment! Practice anything long enough and it becomes reflexive. This applies to our pattern of thoughts as well, and as we've already learned, thoughts are what generate emotions.

We can cultivate the habit of happiness. I was surprised to learn that happy people generally have to work at it; I had thought they were just blessed at birth with the Pollyanna attitude. It was, again, my grandmother, a perpetually kind and happy woman, who explained this to me when she was in her nineties.

In her sweet Southern voice she said, "Honey, when something bad happens, I ask myself, 'Is there anything I can do about it?' And if there is, I do it. Sometimes that'll fix it. Sometimes not. And once there isn't anything else I can do, I tell myself, 'I'm just not going to think about that anymore.' Then I think about things I like. And I crochet or quilt."

She was a master at switching her focus! But she did something more. After she switched her focus, she followed up with some activity that brought her joy. How simple, yet how hard is that to do? Simple, because it's just a matter of changing the track your thought is on (as we already discussed under Switch Your Focus). Hard, because it requires the self-discipline to govern what we think about—the hardest labor of all.

This could not have been easy for my grandmother, either. This was a woman who lived through World War I and the Great Depression, then watched her three sons go off to serve in World War II. She survived three devastating heart attacks in her sixties, and two bouts of breast cancer. She suffered through the death of her youngest son to brain cancer when he was fifty-nine, then the death of her husband of seventy years. Yet here she is, thriving and happy, well past a hundred. What a remarkable testament to the value of doing this work.

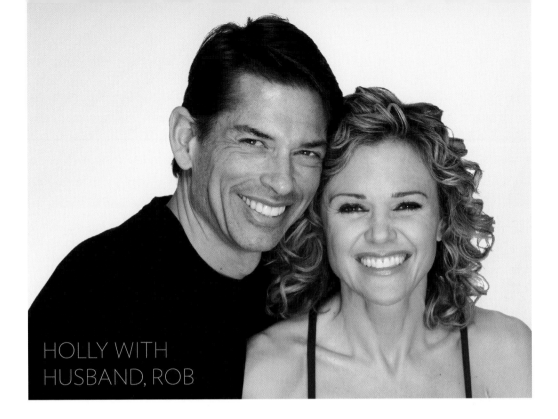

HOLLY WITH
HUSBAND, ROB

CREATE A "HAPPY TASKS" LIST

I work at being happy—not just content, but happy. This goes a step beyond what we learned in Switch Your Focus (page 80). That tool is one I use to bring myself back up to a state of equilibrium, or contentment, when I'm feeling down. I can't just go straight to "happy" from "down in the dumps." I first need to restore myself to equilibrium, then move up the mood scale from there. Happiness is a more elevated mood than contentment. It requires some proactive work, at least for me. So here is what I have found that works.

Take a sheet of paper. Write "Happy Tasks" across the top. Now jot down all the things that make you happy, really happy. For something to make my list, I have to find it worthy of putting a smile on my face or prompting a giggle. Don't think too hard here. You want a stream of consciousness. It can be anything from "take a vacation in Hawaii" to "eat pizza" or "take a bath." From the simple to the sublime, just let it rip.

Now take a look at your list and start to organize it to fit your life. For instance, some of the things on my list are "meditate," "eat frozen yogurt," "take a yoga class," "hike," and "travel to Australia." I ponder and determine how frequently I ideally like to do these things (within reason) to infuse my weeks with good stuff that elevates me to happiness. Then I reorder the list, starting with the things I can easily do and fit into my life and ending with the things that will take time and planning to accomplish but give me something to look forward to.

For instance, based on the five things listed above, my Happy Tasks list will start with (1) meditation (which I need to do every morning to stay happy), then (2) take a yoga class (which I need twice a week), then (3) hike (once a week is ideal), then (4) eat frozen yogurt (I'm good with once a week or once every other week), then finally (5) travel to Australia (which might take more than a year of planning and saving, etc.).

I redo my list every year. I am always open to learning new things and having new experiences, and I find more simple things that make me happy and need to be on my list.

Many times when I find myself in a bit of a funk for no reason, I realize I have skipped out on doing my Happy Tasks from my list. The remedy is easy. I infuse them right back into my weekly schedule, and what do you know? Happy once more.

DEVELOP A
SICK SENSE OF HUMOR

Even if you weren't born with one, you can develop a sense of humor. It starts with making a conscious decision to take a lighter view of life and circumstances and not to take things so seriously. It's all a passing show anyway. Nothing lasts forever. Whether we perceive something that's happened as being wonderful or horrible, one thing is certain: This, too, shall pass. Everything in this life is transitory in nature. So find every excuse you can to laugh.

We can decide to be observers of events, rather than to inject our emotions into every circumstance. As I said before, it's a lot easier to do this when you realize that what you perceive is not necessarily accurate anyway. We don't need to take ourselves so seriously.

If you have a sense of humor that's always at the ready, chances are you will not descend to a negative state of mind quickly or easily. Still, I have found that in spite of my well-developed, sick sense of humor (there is very little I can't laugh about at this point in my life), it's much easier for me to get cranky and negative if I'm tired or operating from a state of depletion—usually because I've overcommitted myself.

So I have my tools to help me laugh. If something happens that is too painful or scary for me to find humor in it, I bring in the big guns. My favorite for several years was my copy of the movie *My Cousin Vinny*. It's hilarious. Being a lawyer, I find this particular movie speaks to me about the sometimes ridiculous things that happen at trial. It never fails to make me laugh, and then I'm on my way back to being positive.

Numerous scientific studies over the past two decades have found that laughter reduces stress, elevates mood, and enhances immunities because it causes the release of dopamine, another feel-good hormone. So humor therapy can work for you too.

I always try to end my day on a positive note, preferably with some laughs. I used to watch the news at night before bed. Big mistake! It was like exposing myself to a toxic dump! So I broke that longtime habit (not an easy habit to break), and now I love watching a comedy show late at night if I'm not sleepy. When I fall asleep with a smile on my face, that mood carries over until morning. I always awaken relaxed and in a great mood.

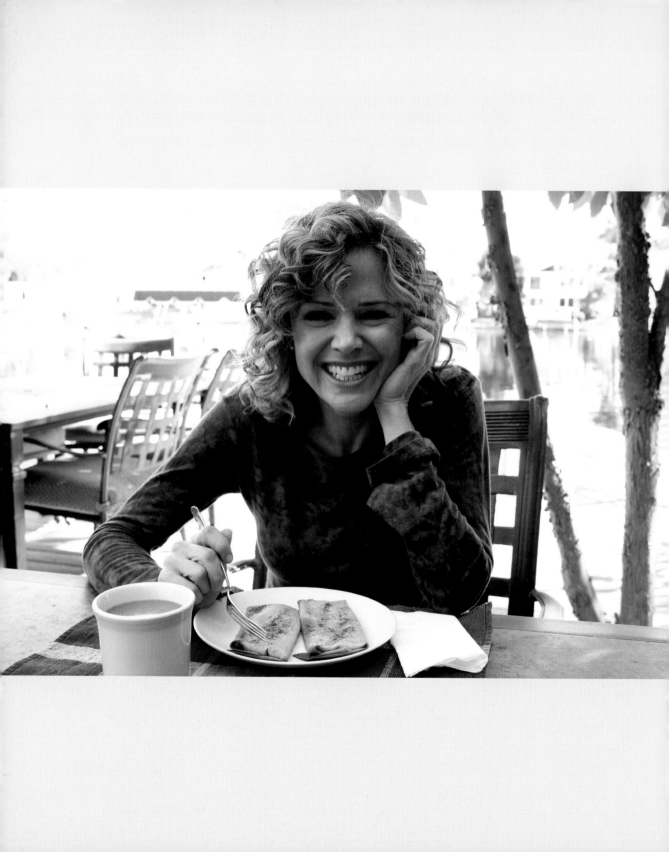

CHAPTER 5

CHOOSE A HAPPIER RESPONSE TO YOUR ENVIRONMENT

As we have discussed, sometimes we have little or no control over the circumstances in which we find ourselves. I don't know about you, but I used to blame my environment for a lot of my stress and unhappiness. I'm not talking about complaining about rain (though in my bleakest days, I did that too), but looking back, I see that many times I focused on the "unfairness" of finding myself in a place I didn't want to be, or involved with events I didn't care about at all.

Some of these situations we can avoid with better planning. That's one of the many benefits of "opting out." You have the time to contemplate and choose what you will participate in and commit to, rather than being railroaded into unnecessary obligations that lack promise for you. But even after we have opted out and have a more peaceful mind and a steadier, calmer approach to life, sometimes we still find ourselves in contrary situations and surroundings. And we all have responsibilities of some sort that, although distasteful, must be carried out.

I developed more tools and techniques to deal with these instances. I may have to physically be in a place where I don't want to be, but I don't have to unwittingly add to the strain by lack of mindfulness and positivity on my part. I never have to mentally succumb to a low level of thought. But for me, with this, as with everything else, I need my little helpers to get me through. They'll help you too.

THE "WHAT DO I LIKE ABOUT IT?" GAME

Years ago, I heard stress defined as "the reaction you have to something that is contrary to what you desire." Isn't that true? I pondered that and realized that stress is the result of our internal resistance to something we don't want. So it occurred to me that if stress is resistance to something unwanted, what if I found something I liked or wanted about the situation? Wouldn't that resolve my stress or at least help reduce it? It made sense to me. So I developed this quick little game that turned out to be *amazingly* effective at counteracting the resistance (stress) that arises in me when I'm confronted with something contrary to what I desire.

Here's how you play. When confronted with anything that causes you to stress, as quickly as you can, ask yourself: "What do I like about it?" Don't edit out any response that comes. This is an internal game, and you play it in your head. So no one is going to know what your answers are to that question. The secrecy is important because it allows you to let go of inhibitions—you don't have to limit your answers to what is politically correct or socially acceptable. For every disaster in life, there is at least a teeny sliver of a silver lining, and by God, this game allows us to find it.

Now, that's important, because this game can very quickly lift you out of "this-is-the-end-of-the-world" catastrophe thinking. Catastrophe thinking is the result of a downward spiral of one negative thought following another, until we reach bottom and find ourselves in complete despair. It's hard to dig our way out from those depths. Instead, I found I can circumvent that whole downward spiral if I intervene with this game. And the earlier I start playing it, the better.

For instance, say a friendship ended, and you are sad. You don't deny your sadness, but you can still ask yourself what you like about not having that particular friendship. Maybe you didn't like that friend's friends so much, and now you won't have to see them anymore. Maybe that friend required a lot of your time, which is now loosened up for you to take an art class, or learn to scuba dive. Maybe you always met that friend for pig-outs, and now you don't have that trigger anymore! (I am laughing at that one, because I had a friendship like that that ended, and I immediately lost five pounds.) In any event, this is your secret mental list, so you can be as outrageous with it as you like. In fact, the more outrageous, the more likely you will start laughing. Once you are laughing, you are healing.

WHAT IF MY SITUATION IS TOO HORRIBLE TO FIND ANYTHING I LIKE ABOUT IT?

We have already seen how the quality of one thought dictates the quality of the thoughts that follow it. So it benefits me, and everyone around me, if I can raise the quality of my thought as soon as possible. And this is true no matter how dire the adverse circumstances appear.

I have read stories about those facing the most horrendous of circumstances and finding a silver lining in their tragedy, then using that little piece as a life preserver. But I was fortunate to meet one of those real-life heroes who faced down a catastrophic diagnosis and joyfully lived on, because although her body was subjected to a terrible illness, her mind was free to go anywhere it wanted. And this lady had the fortitude to guide it to the heights available to us all.

Her name is Annee. She is from Australia (so you can picture her speaking with that lovely accent). Here is her story. In March 1996, at age twenty-five, Annee, then a triathlete, signed up to participate as an amateur crew member in the 2000–2001 BT Global Challenge Round the World Yacht Race. It has been called the world's toughest yacht race. The competition fleet comprises twelve identical yachts. Professional skippers lead crews of amateurs through the world's most treacherous seas over the course of nearly a year. It is, to say the least, grueling.

In July 1998, while undergoing training for the intense race, Annee received devastating news. She was diagnosed with cervical cancer. But that didn't stop her. She started treatment, then checked in for duty on September 10, 2000, with her crew of like-minded adventurists. The race began.

Refusing to wallow in negativity, Annee downplayed her illness and carried out her assigned duties on the yacht. She kept her thoughts moving forward. At each port where they stopped, Annee would disembark for medical checkups and medication changes, then head back to the boat to continue on.

They ran into a hurricane in November 2000, and Annee broke her hand while sailing through it. When her hand didn't heal, she underwent medical tests when her team arrived in Argentina. The tests revealed the cancer was back. She flew to the United Kingdom for more treatment. Then she flew back to the yacht and kept on.

Annee, with her indefatigably buoyant spirit, had the support of not only her crew but the rest of the fleet, to remain on the boat for the remainder of the race. And in spite of the hardships she was undergoing, she found love as well. She met her future husband, Chris, in the midst of all of this. He was a crew member on another one of the yachts.

No matter what happened, Annee disciplined her thought to focus on the positives. She told me of the exhilaration and joy she felt at the sheer thrill of ascending one-hundred-foot waves in the middle of oceans. She related that there was a stillness to be found climbing those monster waves, and she experienced a deep sense of peace there, even as she carried out her multiple duties as a full crew member. The focus required of her helped to keep her mind moving forward, rather than dwelling on the many negatives she could have wallowed in.

In April 2001 she disembarked in South Africa for treatment. While there, she received the most devastating news: Doctors told her she had six months to live, as the cancer had now spread to her brain. In her mind, however, Annee—ever vigilant over her thoughts—decided that no doctor could tell her how long she had to live, and she simply, as she understates it, "carried on."

The race finished in Southampton, England, in June 2001. Annee continued to receive treatment. She married Chris in February 2004, already living past her diagnosis by nearly three years.

Annee went on to continue to learn and thrive, expanding her experiences and developing herself. She learned Chinese medicine and developed a thriving and respected acupuncture practice. She formulated a skin-care line. She continues to travel the world, downplaying her diagnosis (still having to undergo cancer treatments at regular intervals) and focusing, instead, on all the things she can do. She finds what she likes, and although she doesn't call it the "what do I like about it?" game, she naturally lives it.

CRUMBLE OR THRIVE—WE HAVE A CHOICE

Most of us would have fallen apart at such a terrible diagnosis. And who could blame us? But what did Annee do? She exercised discipline over her thoughts and turned to the small sliver of silver lining, and pondered what was still available to her that would bring her joy. The silver lining of her life-threatening diagnosis was that it gave Annee, already an adventurist, the freedom to *really* think outside the box and seriously consider doing things that, under normal circumstances, we probably wouldn't allow ourselves to even think about. And as you can see, there was a lot still available to Annee. She has lived more in the last ten years than many people do in seventy.

I was fortunate to meet Annee and get to spend a week with her in India in the fall of 2010. Annee is now thirty-nine. She was not expected to make it to her thirty-first birthday. She indelibly touched my spirit with her joy—she was more joyous and inspirational than anyone I've met. And few of us are dealing with a diagnosis like hers.

No matter how horrible the circumstance appears, there is a benefit. Just your effort to find even one teeny tiny advantage from it will start to lift your thoughts, and other similar thoughts will start to come. I know, because I do this. And there were many, many times in my past when it seemed that there was absolutely nothing that I could find to like. It can be done. Just ask Annee.

APPLY THE "IS THAT WORTHY OF ME?" TEST

Here's another great little tool to help you weed out unnecessary strain from your life. Ask yourself, "Is that worthy of me?" I apply this test to events, circumstances, entertainment choices, and even friendships. I know where I want my level of consciousness to be, and the higher my state of consciousness, the happier and stress-free I am.

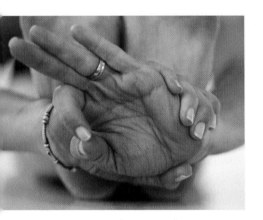

Have you ever seen a ticked-off, stressed-out monk? No. They reside in a tranquillity that I am determined to bring into my typical Western lifestyle. But I have observed how cautious they are about their environment and what they engage with, and I took a lesson from that.

On meditation retreats, there are no TVs or radios—and many times no electronics around whatsoever. The reason is to have a pure environment in which your mind is not being stimulated by unnecessary distractions. In those pristine environments, your mind quiets, and you start to acquaint yourself with your deeper, authentic self, the one we never seem to have access to in our regular lives. (By "pristine environments" I mean they are unencumbered by the regular diversions that usually surround us, like TVs, phones, and so forth. The actual accommodations are usually quite spartan. You cannot believe how soothing that is, once your mind adjusts to it. Such surroundings make the environments filled with "normal" stuff seem noisy!)

In these still, quiet environments is where I find that still, small voice, and it speaks to me, but only in the silence. When I hear it, it is unmistakable and reminds me of those nobler qualities and desires that remain latent behind my human persona. Once I touch that, some of the stuff out here in our culture just seems, well, *icky*. It's like I need to take a shower after being exposed to it.

I don't argue with that anymore. My goal is to reside more and more in these higher levels of consciousness and in the bliss they bring. As studies have confirmed (and we know this anyway), we tend to take on the attributes and attitudes of the people and events we habitually expose ourselves to.

A choice has to be made. I don't want to do the work of raising my level of consciousness only to expose myself to things not worthy of that—and then come tumbling down.

So I ask, internally, is that worthy of me? And by that, I mean my best, deepest me, not the surface ego part of me that comes out to play more often than I'd like.

I have found that holding myself to this standard makes a remarkable difference in lowering my stress. Most of the time we are unaware we are actually choosing to associate with people, events, and things that run counter to our highest goals and loftiest ambitions. It is that crosscurrent that makes us feel like we are swimming upstream much of the time.

I think that is one of the many gifts that aging brings—the awareness that you aren't here forever. I am turning fifty as I write this, and one of the many things I love about getting older is the awareness that I need to get on with creating the life that I want, in every aspect. I no longer languish in that youthful ignorance that tells me I have forever to do anything I want.

This is a good thing. It makes us become more choosy about who and what will populate our life. And when you find your tribe and activities that all support your noblest goals and loftiest ambitions and the best parts of yourself . . . well, I believe that's when you find heaven on Earth.

I know it feels that way to me.

GOVERN YOUR TV AND MOVIE VIEWING

Association brings assimilation. This doesn't apply just to those live humans you hang out with.

What we watch on television or see at the movies has an effect on the quality of our thought. As we've already discussed, our thought governs our emotions and, of course, our actions. A number of studies have found that viewers of snarky-type shows (think of many of the reality shows that stage nasty events to bring out the worst of the cast) act more snarky in their own lives. It makes sense to me. Jealousy and envy are contagious. You can't fill your head with petty grievances and find joy in your life. Yet this is what many of our poor viewing choices have exposed us to.

I know, because I used to watch those shows. I was addicted to the *Real Housewives* series for a while, thinking that seeing others' problems made me feel not so bad about my own. Then I realized that the time I spent filling my head with garbage was not so harmless. At the very least, the time I spent watching it crowded out other, worthwhile activities that would move me closer to my goals. At its worst, it drew me into a negative state of being. Who needs that? And here I was, seeking it out.

Go figure why we do these things. When I step back for even a moment, I am astounded at how easy it is to just mindlessly indulge in something of an unhealthy, and unholy, nature. I don't think any of us would choose to do that if we were alert.

So I am alerting you (and reminding myself!) now. Consciously and carefully pick and choose what you want to view. Resist the urge to even peek at stuff that doesn't support where you want to go or harmonize with the level of consciousness you aspire to have.

This is not to say that TV viewing is bad, or that you should never see a scary movie. Heck, sometimes *South Park* can elevate my thought by making me laugh. What I am saying is to be alert to the effect your viewing choices have on you.

You like vampire shows? Cool. Now ask yourself: How do I feel when I watch them? What desires do they stoke? Do they move me closer to my goals of peace and progress or further away? No show is necessarily bad to watch. Just be alert to what it brings out in you, and if you don't like that, *exercise your self-discipline and don't watch it!*

After I started being selective—very selective—about my viewing choices, I found myself happier all of the time. Remember, moods are contagious, and the mood of the show you watch will catch you. Determine the state of mind you aspire to and select your choices accordingly. You are trading some of your time and precious life energy for access to the show. Make sure it is worthy of you.

DON'T KEEP A MENTAL TALLY

Giving of ourselves is what we were born to do. We are expressive beings, and we naturally share our essence with others. Sometimes things get lopsided. Our efforts and contributions far surpass what we personally derive from whatever it is we are working on.

This used to stress me out. I was raised to work hard. My dad lived through the Great Depression during his formative years, and the lessons he learned about survival were vigorously imprinted on me from my earliest memories. We were taught to work for everything—an exchange of hours of labor for a corresponding allowance. Toys and other luxuries were not just handed over to us; we worked to earn the money to buy these things on our own.

I remember pining for a blue Schwinn bike when I was about nine years old and asking my parents for it as a Christmas gift. Dad told me he admired my great desire, but it was too much for a gift. Instead, he said, increase your chores and I'll up your allowance so you can earn it yourself, and well before Christmas. Deal. I added a few chores to my chore chart with little effort, and that bike was mine within months.

There were so many valuable lessons from being raised in this way. It ultimately gifted me with independence—extending far beyond material things. I learned I could have *anything* I wanted through my own efforts. I am unaware of any way to learn this other than by doing it, and I am afraid my generation has robbed our children of this greatest of all gifts through too much indulgence.

THE DOWNSIDE TO KEEPING A TALLY

There was one downside to this lesson. I trained myself to keep a mental tally of my contributions and to expect a return on my investment. This, of course, is not necessarily a bad thing, but too much of anything creates an imbalance, and we all know the dangers of that. Giving of yourself should not be a quid pro quo—within reason. There are those who give too much and end up depleted, just as there are those who expect something back for any little thing they contribute, whether that takes the form of money or favors. It's the you-scratch-my-back-and-I'll-scratch-yours mentality. Yuck. As with everything else, there is a sweet spot of balance where everyone thrives.

Now, I wasn't mercenary, but I could feel my stress levels rise when I would go through my mental tally of what I had contributed to something that gave me little or no return. I learned two things that resolved this issue for me once and for all.

First, I learned how to say no. I think it was around my forty-fifth birthday that I realized how much precious time and energy I had expended on things that just weren't that important to me. So I began to say no to them, nicely but firmly. I discussed this in more detail earlier in this book under the subheading Opt Out As A Lifestyle.

Saying no to these things instantly lightened my load and reduced my stress. And I saw that one of the reasons I was keeping a mental tally was because when I participated in something that unreasonably strained me, for whatever reason, I couldn't help but feel like I was either paying a debt or buying some peace. This was not a way to find mental equilibrium.

Second, when I chose to participate in something that was meaningful to me, whether with effort or money, I didn't see it so much as a transaction requiring equal give-and-take. In fact, as I observed this over several years, I saw that something magical grew out of sharing myself because I was passionate about something. Instead of being depleted, I was enriched and enlivened in many ways; I just had to lift my gaze a bit. I saw that even if my efforts in one direction did not produce the results I wanted from that specific thing, "unearned" results would crop up from another avenue. It happened again and again.

ALL "LOSSES" CAN FUEL GAINS

Here's an inspiring example of what I am talking about. I recently read an article about the two great female tennis champions Chris Evert and Martina Navratilova. They battled each other at eighty matches, with both of them winning too many championships to list here, but they included eighteen Grand Slam titles for each of them and wins at Wimbledon, the U.S. Open, and the French Open, among many others.

In spite of this professional rivalry, I was surprised to read, they were privately friends. When you are a champion at that level, with all the pressure, joy, and potential devastation that that level of performance brings, who better to go to for comfort than the other person facing the same challenges?

In the article, they were asked what they thought they had that champions need. The answer was not more wins, or an even better record. Instead, Navratilova said it was the "ability to fail. Not being afraid to put it all on the line and come up short. Most people don't have that."[5]

If we peel this back a bit, we see that Navratilova is saying that to be a champion, you must put your full preparation, time, and effort into matches in which someone is going to win and the other is going to lose. And she found those "losses" critical to developing the mental fortitude necessary to win, and win big.

VIEW LIFE AS A WHOLE

If we view life as a whole, rather than dissecting out a single event and placing undue importance on that alone, we can see that all actions bear fruit, whether from the avenue sought or something else. If I stop demanding that my effort in one direction compensate me in some way from that specific thing, the floodgates open and fruit pours in from many different directions.

That's what ceasing the mental tally did for me. It gifted me with an unexpected level of peace. I now feel free to pursue my passions and fully give of myself, knowing that all my efforts will bear fruit somewhere, even if I appear to have lost in the short term. There is no wasted effort.

Try it for yourself. But remember, saying no to stuff that just depletes you is a necessary first step. Then with everything you say yes to, just go for it. Fully participate in the way that makes sense to you, with no mental tally or demand of quid pro quo. Now become very observant, and watch how your efforts in that direction impact seemingly unrelated things in your life, bringing improvement and growth in ways you could not have anticipated. So no more limiting, finite mental tally. Instead, we are exchanging it for an expansive, unlimited view of the circle of life. Peace is found in knowing there is no wasted effort.

What a fun way to go through life!

---

5   Meyers, Kate, "A Winning Friendship," *Parade*, August 29, 2010.

DO WHATEVER WORKS

These chapters just scratch the surface on stress-reduction techniques. There are as many as there are individuals. What I've done is include the main tools that are most effective for me and the people with whom I've shared them. I don't use all of them all of the time, but I do use some of them all of the time—like meditation and focused breathing—because I have found that my daily practice of these two things keeps me in a state of equilibrium at (almost) all times.

But there are countless options out there for you to reduce stress in ways that feel right for you. Once you find the ones that suit you, add them to your arsenal so you always have a stress antidote ready. What you do to relieve stress isn't nearly as important as the fact that you're doing it.

When I incorporate these stress-busters into my life, I feel terrific. Stress lessens, stress hormones dissipate, and I stop battling genuine physical cravings that make weight loss and control an uphill battle, doomed from the start. Now I'm ready to tackle the way I'm eating to optimize my successful weight loss.

In hindsight, if I had to do it all again, I would have dumped the diets. I would have found my favorite stress reducers, quickly worked them into my life in a consistent way, and then and only then would I have revamped the way I was eating. And that doesn't take long! You can enjoy a big reduction in stress in a matter of *days* using the stress-management tools I have given you. Many people tell me they experience tremendous stress relief from the moment they start practicing even one of these marvelous little tools. You'll be quickly primed and ready to revamp those eating habits so the weight starts sliding off. You're gonna love this. It will be the first time you've lost weight with a smile on your face.

It's obvious to me from my vantage point now that my path would have been much easier had I addressed stress before addressing my weight. Oh, well. At least you can benefit from my mistakes. I cleared a path for you, and now you can follow it.

PART TWO

REVAMP THE WAY YOU'RE EATING

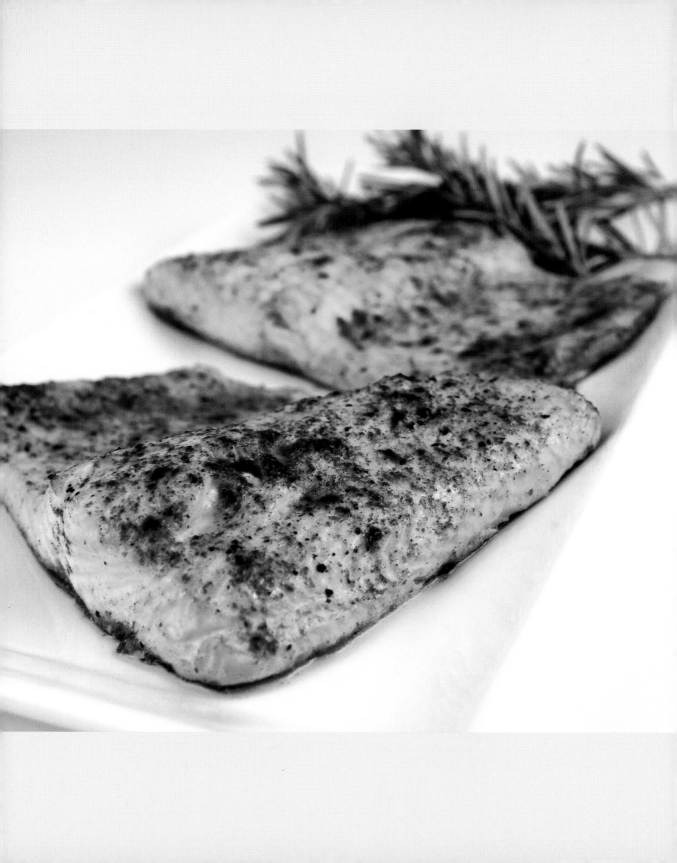

CHAPTER 6

DETERMINE HOW MUCH TO EAT

All those years of battling appetite and cravings, wrestling with control and surrender, working out until I ached, gritting my teeth and struggling to dredge up the willpower to do this . . . If only I had known all those years that it wasn't about willpower at all. It wasn't about fighting or struggling. Once I finally discovered the importance of stress management and harnessed the power of calm, weight control was in my control.

Now that you've learned how to make stress-management techniques a priority in your weight-control plan, you're ready to address the eating plan itself. Without those constant cravings derailing your best intentions, you are better equipped to make intelligent choices about what you put in your body. And now you know that it's not supposed to be a battle. Instead, it's about fully equipping yourself to succeed and setting out on a smarter path.

This chapter is the next step down that path. It sets forth the exact menu guidelines I follow. I developed them during years of research and experimentation. They've given me a level of vigor I hadn't known since childhood. And most important, they allowed me to lose weight and keep it off—easily! What freedom. And these guidelines will help free you too.

I've found that you can lose weight on just about any diet if you take in fewer calories than you expend. There are already countless diets out there, and new ones appear almost daily. And for the most part, they are effective for weight loss. I know, because I tried dozens of diets and lost weight on most of them.

The problem comes in maintaining that weight loss. That's always the real issue, and here's why. Most diets require you to eat in an unnatural manner. They require unusual foods, complicated recipes with exotic ingredients, or the relinquishment of your favorite foods. They require you to eat in a way that makes you eat separate meals from those your family eats, because your kids just aren't going for all-natural, all-raw, no-sugar, or no-dairy meals. They require you to omit entire food groups. They require you to purchase meals in a box. They require you to do all sorts of artificial things that you couldn't possibly sustain for the rest of your life. And when you stop doing them and go back to your previous way of eating—or any other eating pattern that feels normal and natural to you—you gain the weight back.

But people who have followed my plan report the same results I have enjoyed: increased energy, easy weight loss eating the foods they love, and effortless maintenance. Why do they get this result? The same reason I do: because this way of eating isn't unnatural, complex, or extraordinary. It's easy to follow. It includes regular foods your whole family enjoys. The recipes are quick and simple and they use five ingredients or fewer, for the most part. Best of all, they use stuff that you already have in your pantry.

My plan allows you to go to restaurants. It recognizes that it's just too darned hard to stick with an contrived eating regimen that requires you to shop for exotic ingredients, make complex recipes, give up the foods you love—in short, makes you look forward to the day when you reach your weight-loss goal so you can just get off of that diet!

PICK YOUR "HAPPY WEIGHT"

Okay, it's decision time. What is the right weight for you? The ideal weight varies widely from one person to the next, even for people with similar height and bone structure. One person's satisfaction at 145 pounds is another's despair over being too big. And there's nothing wrong with that.

Contrary to the wise words of our forefathers, we were not all created equal. We were created as individuals, and that's wonderful! What makes you laugh may not get me to crack a smile. My favorite foods may taste like garbage to you. If every woman were built like Marilyn Monroe, then she wouldn't seem so special. And of course Twiggy was a different kind of beauty. Without all this variety, the world would be infinitely less interesting.

Yet in our culture we are trained to force ourselves into the mold formed by those who've gone before us. We chase after an ideal that may or may not be achievable for each of us. And we can learn vast amounts from those ideals, but the wisdom we need develops only when we meld what we observe of others with solid knowledge of what works perfectly for us. And what works perfectly for us is always an outgrowth of our personal life path—a path that's ours alone.

We can choose to recognize and honor our own preferences, or we can choose instead to beat ourselves into fitting a mold others have formed. It's up to us. But when we honor and follow our personal preferences, then we have something of true value to contribute and share with others.

I choose 107 to 108 pounds as my "happy weight." I am five feet two inches and small-boned. My body doesn't carry excess weight well, and this is the weight that feels best on my tiny frame. Besides that, as I progressed in yoga, I wanted to fly—and that's much easier for me when I'm lighter.

I'm convinced that for most of us, our happy weight stems from the other things in life that we associate with it. My happy weight is a wonderful reminder of a stimulating time in my life when I was an actress, striving to succeed, with all the joy and excitement that dreaming big brings. So 107 to 108 it was—for me.

But it may not be for you, even if you're five feet two. Maybe 130 pounds is your happy weight. That's fine. The only rule to apply here is that you should choose a weight that is medically sound and healthy. Nothing good can come of an adult who is five feet eight inches and striving to weigh 105 pounds. That's a faulty foundation on which to build any program.

How do you choose a happy weight that is medically sound and healthy? A good place to start is by asking your regular doctor for input. That's a good safety measure because your doctor will take into account your blood pressure and cholesterol levels, any issues with your blood sugar (like whether you are headed for or have diabetes), or if you have or are at risk for cardiovascular disease at your current weight.

But generally, if all of these things are normal (and it's good to confirm that they are before starting any type of fitness plan), doctors just follow medical charts that list a fairly expansive acceptable weight range per height. For example, according to medical charts I've seen, my "acceptable weight range" goes from 108 to 143 pounds, depending on whether I am small-, medium-, or large-boned! (And as I have said, I am small-boned.)

Within a medically acceptable weight range, how do you choose? The Hamwi formula is a generally accepted formula to help you choose your happy weight. It is just a guideline, not gospel. But I think it is a useful place to start.

For women, the Hamwi formula allows 100 pounds for the first five feet. Then you add five pounds for each inch over five feet. For small-framed individuals, subtract approximately 10 percent. For large-framed individuals, add approximately 10 percent.

For men, the Hamwi formula allows 106 pounds for the first five feet, and six pounds for each inch over five feet. For small-framed individuals, subtract 10 percent. For large-framed individuals, add 10 percent.

The next question is, What is your frame size? That is determined by your wrist circumference in relation to your height.

For women: if you are under five feet two inches, a small frame is a wrist measurement of less than five and one-half inches, a medium frame is a wrist measurement of five and one-half to five and three-quarters inches, and a large frame is more than five and three-quarters inches. If you are five feet two to five feet five inches, a small frame is a wrist measurement of less than six inches, medium is a wrist measurement of six to six and one-quarter inches, and large is more than six and one-quarter inches. For women over five feet five inches, a small frame is a wrist measurement of less than six and one-quarter inches, medium is a wrist size of six and one-quarter to six and one-half inches, and large is more than six and one-half inches.

For men there is a more general rule: if you are taller than five feet five inches, a small frame is a wrist measurement of five and one-half to six and one-half inches, a medium frame is a wrist measurement of six and one-half to seven and one-half inches, and a large frame is more than seven and one-half inches.

Let's take a look at this. According to the Hamwi formula, my base weight at five feet two is 110. But I am small-boned. So according to this, I subtract 10 percent, or eleven pounds. That would put me at 99 pounds! (Too skinny for me.) But I do feel best at around 107 to 108, so a slight reduction from 110 feels right (and very good) to me.

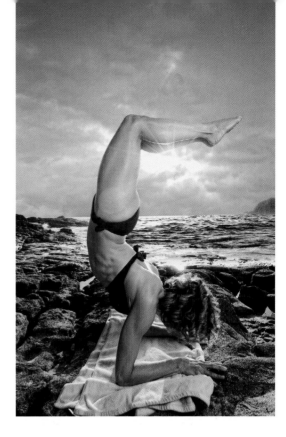

And that's how you choose. You apply the formulas to get an idea, not an exact answer. You won't find a formula that can determine your ideal body weight accurately, anyway. We have too many differences in bone structure, frame size, and percentage of fat and muscle to allow any one formula to provide an exact answer. So determine your range using these formulas I've given you, then pick what feels right for you within that range. Like the name implies, you want this to be your "happy" weight, not a tortured weight!

We're seeking health and vitality here, not perpetuating dysfunction. Be willing to come clean with yourself and become aware of your reasons for the happy weight you choose. I have found that once you reach that awareness, it releases a mountain of old emotional garbage and allows you to begin this journey forward on a light and positive note. And I believe that like attracts like, so this is all good and has wonderful ramifications well beyond just the number on your scale.

By the way, your happy weight can change to reflect your personal growth. If you begin to feel better at 120 pounds, even though you used to use 110 as your personal ideal, that's okay. Within the boundaries of medical safety, your happy weight need only be the one at which you feel healthy, energetic, and fit.

LEARN THE CORRECT DAILY CALORIE ALLOTMENT TO REACH YOUR HAPPY WEIGHT

Most people have no idea how many calories they consume, much less how many they should aim for to lose weight. Most of the time we vastly underestimate the number of calories we eat. I was shocked when I actually began to calculate my daily caloric average by measuring every food I ate. I estimated that I was getting about 1,500 calories per day. My homework uncovered that I was actually consuming a whopping 2,600 calories. That's a big difference!

There are no magic bullets or mystical elixirs that will allow us to avoid the truth: To lose weight, we must consume fewer calories than we burn. Bummer! But when you follow the eating guidelines that I give you in the next chapters, you'll find this is a heck of a lot easier than the tormented process that you've likely experienced in the past. In fact, I'm willing to bet you will have the same experience that I did—it will be hard for you to believe you are eating fewer calories than you used to because you will feel more satiated on fewer calories . . . if you follow my plan.

To determine how many calories you should eat each day to reach your happy weight, look at the Approximate Daily Calorie Consumption charts that follow.

That will give you a good estimate. Or, if you have access to the Internet, you can visit my website at www.hollymosier.com. I have a really cool tool there to calculate the daily calories needed to reach your goal weight.

A word of warning: Give yourself *plenty* of time to lose the weight. You want to pace it at a pound or two per week. You want a slow, steady, and safe weight loss that allows your body and mind to acclimate successfully to the new and healthier way of eating and to build new and better habits.

You need your body and your mind to work harmoniously to have permanent results, and a quick fix does not allow for this. It takes time to form new habits of any kind. A quick fix feels foreign on many levels, and once you hit your goal, you'll go back to the old and familiar ways of eating. It's human nature to seek familiarity, because it feels safe.

If you ease into this new pattern, it will begin to feel comfortable and normal to you. After a few weeks, your old eating style will begin to feel foreign. That's worth celebrating, because it means that the results you achieve will more likely be permanent.

A multitude of studies have confirmed that this slow and steady approach is by far the most successful for permanent weight loss. There are all sorts of reasons why this is true. To lose weight quickly, you must generally decrease your normal calorie consumption severely. Although you may get a short psychological boost from the fast results, it won't last. Obesity studies have found that people typically consumed 700 fewer calories the day before a binge. In other words, you're setting yourself up for failure by putting your body in deprivation mode.

Your normal eating habits aren't erased overnight. They need time to fade and eventually get replaced with the new, healthier patterns. It's not helpful at all to rush the process as if you're simply changing channels on the television. Allow your mind and body a little time to adjust to the new pattern. It does happen, and it happens much more successfully if you approach the process with compassion and give your body some time to catch up.

I know this slow-and-steady approach is not a popular one. Our fast-food culture has trained us to expect instant gratification. Once we decide to lose weight, we want it to happen this second. And if you've ever dieted before (of course you have!), you know that many diet plans and products prey on this desire. Whatever we want, we want it *now*. But if there's one thing I've learned through personal experience and by observing others over decades, it's this: The quicker you lose the weight, the quicker you gain it back.

And let me just say a word here about weight-loss programs that make outrageous claims like "Lose ten pounds a week!" I know that sounds good, but to lose just one pound of *fat* (not just water weight) per week, you must burn 500 calories more than you took in every day. To lose two pounds of fat per week, you must burn

APPROXIMATE DAILY CALORIE CONSUMPTION
RECOMMENDED **FOR AN AVERAGE WOMAN**

Weight (in pounds)	Sedentary	Light Activity	Moderate Activity	High Activity
100	1390	1590	1800	2000
110	1450	1660	1870	2080
120	1500	1720	1940	2160
130	1550	1780	2010	2240
140	1610	1840	2080	2320
150	1660	1910	2150	2390
160	1720	1970	2220	2470
170	1770	2030	2290	2550
180	1830	2090	2360	2630
190	1880	2150	2430	2710
200	1940	2220	2500	2780
210	1990	2280	2570	2860
220	2040	2340	2640	2940
230	2100	2400	2710	3020
240	2150	2470	2780	3090
250	2210	2530	2850	3170
260	2260	2590	2920	3250
270	2320	2650	2990	3330
280	2370	2720	3060	3410
290	2430	2780	3130	3490
300	2480	2840	3200	3560
310	2530	2900	3270	3640
320	2590	2970	3340	3720
330	2640	3030	3410	3800
340	2700	3090	3480	3880
350	2750	3150	3550	3960

APPROXIMATE DAILY CALORIE CONSUMPTION
RECOMMENDED **FOR AN AVERAGE MAN**

Weight (in pounds)	Sedentary	Light Activity	Moderate Activity	High Activity
100	1690	1930	2180	2420
110	1740	1990	2250	2500
120	1790	2060	2320	2580
130	1850	2120	2390	2660
140	1900	2180	2460	2740
150	1960	2240	2530	2810
160	2010	2310	2600	2890
170	2070	2370	2670	2970
180	2120	2430	2740	3050
190	2180	2490	2810	3130
200	2230	2550	2880	3200
210	2280	2620	2950	3280
220	2340	2680	3020	3360
230	2390	2740	3090	3440
240	2450	2800	3160	3520
250	2500	2870	3230	3590
260	2560	2930	3300	3670
270	2610	2990	3370	3750
280	2670	3050	3440	3830
290	2720	3120	3510	3910
300	2770	3180	3580	3990
310	2830	3240	3650	4070
320	2880	3300	3720	4140
330	2940	3370	3790	4220
340	2990	3430	3860	4300
350	3050	3490	3930	4380

1,000 calories more than you took in every day. To lose three pounds of fat per week, you must have a calorie deficit of 1,500 per day. So to really lose ten pounds in a week (I'm talking real fat here, not just water weight), you would have to have a 5,000-calorie deficit *per day*! That's impossible—or at least impossible to achieve in any kind of balanced and healthy manner.

That's why I think the best, healthiest, and most solid plan for *permanent* results is to follow my above recommendations and aim to lose a pound or two per week. I know that will sound slow to many of you, but it *works*.

Your goal is to exit the diet roller coaster once and for all. So be patient with yourself. You didn't gain the weight in a day or a week or a month. Even if you could take it off that quickly, a rebound would be virtually inevitable. This time, give yourself the time to do it right.

DIVVY UP YOUR DAILY CALORIES AMONG BREAKFAST, LUNCH, DINNER, AND A SNACK

When I know how many calories I'm allowed for each meal and snack, it's much easier to stay within my daily allotment. It breaks up the day into smaller goals that are easier to achieve. When I started, I initially divided my daily number to match the way I am normally inclined to eat. If you tend to eat less at breakfast and more at dinner, then divide your daily calories into amounts that reflect that. If you're a healthy adult, there's no reason this shouldn't work for you.

I know there are many experts who recommend getting the majority of your calories earlier in the day. This is probably good advice, but it has never worked for me. I am just naturally not that hungry early in the day. Forcing myself to eat when I'm not hungry made me lethargic and, frankly, *hungrier* throughout the day! But it works for my husband, and it may work for you. Keep it in mind as you're formulating your own personal plan.

So here's how I did it. At my activity level, I need 1,700 to 1,800 calories per day to stay at 107 to 108 pounds, my happy weight. Because I am almost never hungry in the morning, I allot myself about 350 calories for breakfast. (Research has consistently shown that people who skip breakfast tend to gain more weight and have a harder time keeping weight off. So although I would generally rather skip breakfast, I don't.)

I'm usually still not really hungry at lunch, so I allot myself about 450 calories. I like to eat some plain fruit in the late afternoon, so I allot 100 calories for this snack. That leaves me with about 800 to 900 calories for dinner, and maybe a little bite of dessert.

Because this allotment follows my natural hunger patterns, it has been easy for me to do. I rarely feel hungry; nor do I ever feel shaky, as if my blood sugar has dropped too low. I feel vigorous and energetic throughout the day.

I can also mix it up if I want. If I go to a restaurant for lunch, I may choose to switch it around and eat less for dinner in exchange for splurging a bit at lunch. But because I always know how many calories are available for each meal, it's easy to make changes without inadvertently overeating. I simply eat my 800 or 900 calories for lunch and about 450 at dinner. Simple.

You can carve up your daily calorie allotment to suit your own needs. You don't have to follow the way I divided mine to get the results you're after. You may want two snacks a day. Some people, like my friend Jen, like to eat every three hours. That's fine. Adjust your plan accordingly, and experiment a little. See how you feel after each meal and snack, and make revisions as needed. The most important thing is to know how many calories you have available each time you eat.

If you have a medical condition such as diabetes or hypoglycemia, or if you take certain medications, you'll need to consult your doctor as to how to mete out your daily calories and maintain a consistent blood sugar level. Bring this book to your doctor for help on accommodating your medical needs. My plan will work for everyone. Just make sure you follow your doctor's instructions.

You've chosen what you want to weigh, and now you know how many calories a day you can have to reach your goal. But this needs to be an easy, enjoyable lifestyle change that you'll maintain so you will never again feel the despair of zippers that just won't go up. I've found the magic formula for ways of eating that will bring you to your goal without struggle and strain. Read on—your days of trading comfort for being slim are over!

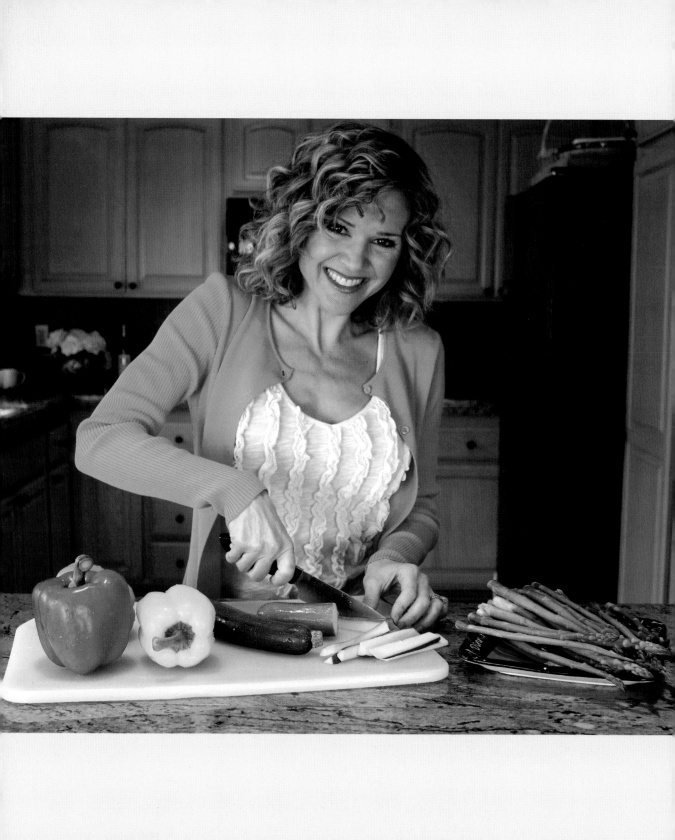

CHAPTER 7

MAKE THE RIGHT DECISIONS ABOUT WHAT TO EAT

I've learned that when it comes to losing weight in a comfortable manner, where you are not starving and ready to eat the curtains off the rods, not all foods are created equal. I found (and I'm sure you have too) that just because a food is nutritious, it isn't necessarily satiating. But after a lot of experimentation, I discovered that if I ate nutritious foods in certain combinations, I was easily satiated. With these new, informed choices about what to eat, I wasn't constantly thinking about food and longing for my next meal for the first time in my life. That's when the weight started to slide off. It was so easy, I could not believe the numbers on the scale were on a downward descent. Welcome to my little secrets!

BALANCE THE CARBOHYDRATES, PROTEINS, AND FATS IN YOUR MEALS

I am a carb lover. Give me some frozen yogurt, a bran muffin, or a plate of spaghetti, and I am a happy camper. I happily ate an almost-all-carb diet for most of my life, and I didn't run into problems until my forties, when midlife hormonal changes forced me to examine how the same foods I had been eating for years were starting to cause me to gain weight and suffer tremendous fatigue.

Using the information I learned from dozens of studies, I grudgingly decided to reduce my carbohydrate intake a bit and start adding some protein to my meals, as well as a little more fat.

HIGH-CARB EATING WAS CAUSING ME PROBLEMS

According to my research, my high-carbohydrate eating style was causing several of my problems. First, significant variations in blood sugar levels throughout the day were likely one of the culprits of my big appetite spikes, contributing to my weight gain. Second, high carbohydrate intake elicits increased insulin secretions, and this insulin boost was causing me to retain water. Last, but truly not least, I suffered from overwhelming fatigue. Again, the swings in blood sugar throughout the day were big contributors to the problem. Also, the water retention triggered many nightly visits to the bathroom. These constant sleep interruptions wreaked havoc on my energy levels all day long.

I also learned from my research that protein takes longer to digest than carbohydrates do, and it helps stabilize blood sugar levels. That means you won't get hungry again so soon after eating. Fat—another component I was neglecting—helps us to feel satiated, and we need it to assimilate the nutrients in our foods.

My food journal helped me with the math. I quickly determined that whenever the meal I ate comprised roughly 40 percent carbohydrates, 30 to 35 percent protein, and about 25 to 30 percent fat, I felt great. I was satiated and energetic, and furthermore, I felt a lot less hungry than I did when I was eating many more calories per day in the form of my beloved carbs.

This calculation is not at all precise; it's a rough estimate. So don't worry—you won't need to enroll in a nutrition class to ensure you're having exactly 40 percent carbohydrates at every meal. Just strive for the above ratios as guidelines for each meal by including a carbohydrate, a protein, and a fat source.

CARBS/PROTEINS/FATS CHART

CARBS	CARBS/PROTEINS	PROTEINS	FAT
Breads	Milk	Fish	Butter
Bagels	Cottage Cheese	Poultry	Oils
Cereal	Ricotta	Meat	Lard
Pasta	Yogurt	Cheese	
Beans	Protein Bars	Eggs	
Rice	Nuts		
Veggies	Peanut Butter		
Fruit			
Sugars			

Let me give you some examples of how I apply these ratios. Before I developed these guidelines, I used to eat a bran muffin or a whole-grain bagel with cream cheese for breakfast. That's almost all carbs with a little fat. Now I'll have only half the bagel or muffin and add two eggs—a good source of protein and fat. So my breakfasts today are more balanced.

For lunch, I used to go for fruit and yogurt (which is nutrient-rich but higher in sugar and carbs than in protein and contains almost no fat) or a baked potato (all carbs). Now, if I have yogurt, I'll start with two low-fat string cheeses or almonds (lots of protein and some fat) instead of the fruit. If I have a baked potato, I'll eat only half and pair it with a lean protein, like a chicken breast, or even low-fat cottage cheese.

A typical dinner I used to eat was spaghetti and salad, or veggies and rice, sometimes with a glass of wine—almost all carbs. Now, I still have the spaghetti and salad or the veggies and rice (and a small glass of wine), but I eat smaller portions of the spaghetti and rice and add some beef or turkey meatballs or a piece of fish for some protein and fat.

YES, YOU CAN STILL HAVE A DRINK ON THE PLAN

You don't have to give up any food or drink you love to be successful on this plan, and I certainly don't. I am a wine lover, and there is no way I'm cutting it out. But I will be smart about it. Wine and other alcoholic beverages count as carbs, or starch, and they contain significant calories. For example, most wines are about 120 calories for four ounces. Four ounces of wine is a pretty small glass. Most hard liquor is about 65 to 80 calories per ounce, and that doesn't include the calories in the mixer.

So there are three things to do if you are including wine or alcohol with your meal: (1) make sure to include the calories from it in your calorie count for that meal; (2) if you are drinking hard alcohol, mix it with a low- or no-calorie mixer, like diet cola, diet tonic, or club soda; and (3) skip or minimize the starch with your meal. Substitute a larger portion of green salad or low-glycemic (non-starchy) veggie for bread, potatoes, rice, corn, or peas.

LOOK AT NUTRITION LABELS OR GO TO THE WEB

Some foods' nutrition labels tell you how many grams of carbohydrates, protein, and fat they contain. That makes it easier to determine your ratios. But again, I have found that you need not be meticulous with the percentages. Just be sure to add protein to every meal. (For ideas, take a look at the protein-rich foods in the Carbs/Proteins/Fats Chart on page 121.)

FRESH IDEA: *One of my favorite high-protein foods is low-fat cottage cheese. I keep it stocked in my refrigerator because of its versatility. At about 160 calories per cup, you can eat it by itself if you want, for a high-protein meal. (I mix it with cinnamon and Splenda for a delicious breakfast.) Or you can add it as a side dish to boost the protein content of just about any meal. (I think it goes great with a burger patty and a salad. I even add it to my spaghetti if I don't have meatballs on hand.)*

What if you don't have a nutrition label to guide you? What if you're eating a fresh food that doesn't come in a package? I check Web sites like www.thedailyplate.com, www.calorieking.com, and www.calorie-count.com to get an idea of how much carb, protein, and fat a food contains.

Eventually, you are going to have to eyeball a portion size. Roll up your sleeves and use your hands—literally.

- A protein portion should be about the size of the palm of your hand.
- A starch or carb portion should take about half the volume of your balled-up fist.
- Your thumb shows you the maximum fat and oil you should have in a single meal. But be careful, especially at restaurants. There is a lot of hidden fat in foods, so always cut away visible fat. (For example, take the skin off your grilled chicken.)

You're always safest if you have a plan. The heat of the moment is no time to make tough decisions. That's why I try to plan my food the night before. If I know I'm going to have a carb-heavy dinner (like pasta) the next night, I try to eat a higher-protein lunch (for example, a piece of fish and a salad and no bread). It's always much easier for me to follow my plan, rather than try to choose wisely once I'm already hungry.

ABOVE ALL ELSE, GET ADEQUATE PROTEIN IN YOUR BREAKFAST

I am frequently asked if I have one piece of advice I believe is most important for weight loss. And I do. If I were to implement only one of my guidelines, it would be to make sure I got adequate protein in my breakfast every single day.

Why? Giving up my glorious almost-all-carb breakfasts and adding protein reduced my voracious appetite and debilitating fatigue. I no longer got that blood sugar "high" we get as carbs are metabolized, followed by the crash that would send me to bed for a daily nap. And my appetite stayed in check all day.

You'll notice all-carb breakfasts are common. Most morning business meetings include bagels, croissants, or donuts, sometimes with some fruit (also a carb). Hotels frequently offer a continental breakfast—typically some kind of bread and orange juice (carbs and sugar). Most breakfast gatherings are carb-fests.

I enter these situations prepared. I pack some protein in my purse or briefcase—two hard-boiled eggs, a couple of pieces of low-fat string cheese, a protein bar, or some almonds. There's always coffee or tea served at these gatherings, so it's easy for me to get my hot beverage (see p. 133), and I can still have half a bagel or whatever other carb I choose.

CHOOSE LOWER-GLYCEMIC FOODS

The glycemic index (GI) measures the effect a food has on your blood sugar level. It ranges from zero to one hundred, and the higher the GI rating, the higher and faster that food causes your blood sugar level to rise. What goes up must come down. This "spike and crash syndrome," as it is called, sparks appetite.

You can check where a food rates on the glycemic index on the chart on pages 126–127. If you have access to the Internet, you can find the glycemic index on many Web sites. I generally use the University of Sydney's Web site, www.glycemicindex.com or www.lowglycemicdiet.com, but there are many others. The information is easy to find in book form as well.

A rating of fifty-five or under is "low" on the GI. Simply put, foods that rate "low" have a more stabilizing effect on the blood sugar level. Generally, low-GI foods are high-fiber, unprocessed foods, such as most fresh fruits and vegetables. Whole-grain foods, such as whole-grain breads and pastas, are also low on the GI, as are many dairy products, such as milk and low-fat cottage cheese.

A rating of fifty-six to sixty-nine is considered "medium." Generally, starchier vegetables and sweeter fruits fall in this range, like corn, raisins, and baked sweet potatoes (which, surprisingly, have a lower GI than regular baked russet potatoes).

A "high" GI rating is seventy or above. Certain carbohydrates, especially starchy, sugary, and processed carbs (products containing white sugar and white flour) rate high on the GI. A doughnut rates at around seventy-six. A piece of white bread rates seventy-one. Instant white rice rates eighty-seven. Pretzels are eighty-one. Many sugary sports drinks also rate high—very high. But there are some healthy fresh foods that rate high as well, such as watermelon, which rates seventy-two.

On the other end of the scale, foods that have no carbohydrate content have no GI rating, or are sometimes said to have a GI rating of zero (like beef, fish, and cheese). A zero rating means the food has little effect on the blood sugar level. In essence, it helps blood sugar levels remain steady.

Keep your blood sugar off the blood sugar roller coaster and its dangerous appetite fluctuations. Try to eat most of your foods from the low end of the GI scale, rating fifty-five or under. It's not that you shouldn't eat foods that rate higher. Some, liked baked russet potatoes, corn, and cantaloupe, are very nutritious. But eat them alongside foods with much lower GI ratings, and you can avoid the appetite spikes that can derail your daily eating plan.

For example, enjoy your high-GI baked potato with a chicken breast or pork chop. Eat cantaloupe with a meal that includes eggs or some other protein and fat. Spread some peanut butter (a low-GI food that's filled with heart-healthy good fat) on your higher-GI toast.

You can lower the GI rating of your meal by balancing in this way—offsetting a medium- or high-GI food with either a low-GI food or a pure protein, like chicken, that has no GI rating because it contains no carbs.

Occasionally you'll still opt for the high-GI meal or snack. Not to worry. British researchers in one study found that participants who consumed twelve ounces of hot black tea after a meal lowered their postmeal blood sugar levels significantly.[6] So go ahead and indulge occasionally. Then, drink up!

ADD CINNAMON TO YOUR FOODS, IF POSSIBLE

Several studies have found that half a teaspoon of cinnamon a day can significantly reduce blood sugar levels. And there's another benefit—other studies have shown it also lowers "bad" or LDL cholesterol.

---

6   Bryans, Judith A., Patricia A. Judd, and Peter R. Ellis, "The Effect of Consuming Instant Black Tea on Postprandial Plasma Glucose and Insulin Concentrations in Healthy Humans," *Journal of the American College of Nutrition*, Volume 26, No. 5 (2007), 471–477.

GLYCEMIC INDEX

GLYCEMIC INDEX: Low: 55 and under ■ Medium: 56 to 69 ■ High: 70 and above					
Fruits					
Cherries	Low	22	Grapefruit	Low	25
Apricots (dried)	Low	31	Strawberries/Berries	Low	32
Apples	Low	38	Pears	Low	38
Plums	Low	39	Peaches	Low	42
Oranges	Low	44	Grapes	Low	46
Bananas	Low	54			
Mangoes	Medium	56	Apricots	Medium	57
Raisins	Medium	64	Pineapple	Medium	64
Watermelon	High	72	Dates	High	103
Vegetables and Beans					
Cabbage	Low	10	Onions	Low	10
Artichoke	Low	15	Asparagus	Low	15
Broccoli	Low	15	Cauliflower	Low	15
Celery	Low	15	Cucumber	Low	15
Eggplant	Low	15	Green beans	Low	15
Lettuce, all varieties	Low	15	Peppers, all varieties	Low	15
Snow peas	Low	15	Spinach	Low	15
Squash	Low	15	Tomatoes	Low	15
Zucchini	Low	15	Kidney beans	Low	29
Lentils, green	Low	29	Black-eyed beans	Low	41
Carrots, raw	Low	47	Yam	Low	51
Sweet potato	Medium	56			
Potato, new	Medium	57	Potato, mashed	Medium	70
Carrots, cooked	High	71	Potato chips	High	75
Potato, instant	High	83	Potato, russet, baked	High	85
Parsnips	High	97			

Breads					
Multigrain bread	Low	48	Whole grain	Low	50
Pita bread, white	Medium	57	Pizza, cheese	Medium	60
Hamburger bun	Medium	61	Rye-flour bread	Medium	64
Whole-wheat bread	Medium	69			
White bread	High	71	White rolls	High	73
Baguette	High	95			
Cereal					
Bran cereals	Low	42	Oatmeal	Low	49
Kellogg's All-Bran	Low	51	Kellogg's Special K	Low	54
Oat bran	Medium	55	Mini-Wheats	Medium	55
Shredded Wheat	Medium	69			
Golden Grahams	High	71	Puffed wheat	High	74
Dairy					
Yogurt, low-fat	Low	14	Milk, chocolate	Low	24
Milk, whole	Low	27	Milk, skim	Low	32
Milk, 2%	Low	34	Ice cream (low-fat)	Low	50
Ice cream	Medium	61			
Snacks					
Peanuts	Low	15	M&M's (peanut)	Low	33
Snickers bar	Low	40	Chocolate bar, 30 g	Low	49
Jelly/Jam	Low	49			
Popcorn	Medium	55	Mars bar	Medium	64
Table sugar	Medium	65			
Corn chips	High	74	Jelly beans	High	80
Pretzels	High	81			

Anytime you are eating a high-GI or high-sugar food, try sprinkling some cinnamon on it, or put some in your coffee or tea. You don't need a lot. According to researchers, the cinnamon will help keep your blood sugar level from rapidly elevating and help prevent that "spike and crash syndrome" associated with high-carb, high-sugar meals and snacks.

Many mornings I have cottage cheese with Splenda and cinnamon so I can take advantage of this benefit. It seems to "set" my blood sugar for the rest of the day.

EAT HIGH-VOLUME, LOW-GLYCEMIC FOODS AT THE BEGINNING OF THE MEAL

We're hungriest when we first sit down to eat, and we're inclined to attack the densest foods first. When I'm really hungry, I'll naturally eat the slice of pizza before the salad. The problem with this approach is that it takes time to register that we're full. By the time your stomach has sent your brain the signals that you're full, you may have actually overeaten. Even worse, within twenty minutes, you're stuck with that uncomfortably full feeling. (And maybe you'll regret eating three slices of pizza before even picking at the salad.)

Train yourself to begin meals with the higher-volume, lower-glycemic foods. Then eat your protein, and save carbohydrates for last. The salad and veggies will begin to fill you up so that you're less likely to overeat the more calorie-dense proteins and carbs. People who eat this way eat about 12 percent fewer calories per meal, according to some studies. Other studies indicate the same can be true for those who start the meal with a broth-based soup. It's the same idea—you start filling your stomach with high-volume, low-calorie food, so you'll eat less of the other stuff.

I'm not a big fan of soup, but I get the same effect by having a hot beverage with my meals. I think I get a double bang for my buck when I drink something hot with my daily salad at the beginning of my meal. Give this a try and see how it works for you.

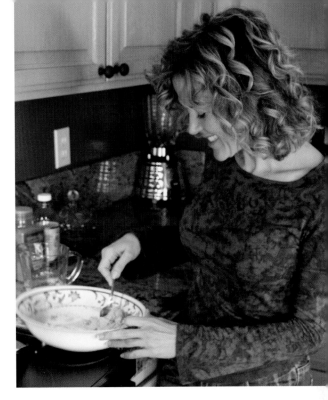

It's much easier than it might sound. I start almost every dinner with either Holly's Salad or Holly's Roasted Veggies (you'll find these easy recipes in Chapter Twelve). If I pair the veggies or salad with hot tea (or water or iced tea . . .), I'm already starting to get satiated before I get to my higher-density, higher-calorie chicken—my protein. Although I might have a few bites of rice with my chicken, I'll generally save most of the carbs for last. And because I'm no longer "starving" by the time I eat the rice, it's a heck of a lot easier to eat a proper portion and not load up on seconds (or thirds).

When I eat this way, I rarely end up with that awful bursting-at-the-seams full feeling because my brain catches up with what I'm putting in my body and starts sending me "you're getting full" signals by the time I get to my higher-density, higher-calorie foods.

Try it and see how it feels.

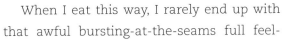

DON'T EAT TOO MUCH VARIETY

Studies have found that naturally thin people tend not to eat a huge variety of foods. They stick to a fairly predictable menu. Why does this help with weight control? Researchers believe this regularity of foods prevents slim people from being tempted to overindulge. The greater the variety of foods on our plate—lots of tastes and textures—the more likely it is we will eat more, hungry or not.

If you think about it, it makes sense. How hard is it to avoid overeating at a buffet? Or at a party where they're serving lots of tasty appetizers? And we always seem to have room for dessert, no matter how full we are. All that selection triggers a feeding frenzy as the brain signals us to eat the "new" food in front of us.

This isn't to say you should eat the same foods day after day. You can still enjoy some variety, and you should, because different foods contain different essential nutrients. I don't eat the same foods every day, or the same dinners on the same days of the week. But I don't load my plate with six or seven different selections—I'll have my salad, veggies, and one entrée, instead of sampling several entrées.

I've picked my favorite foods that meet my guidelines, and those compose the majority of my weekly menu. Plus, it makes it a heck of a lot easier to shop for groceries.

I bet that using these suggestions have already brought your appetite more under control and allowed you to make intelligent choices about what you are eating. But more help is on the way. Read on for some more pointers about what you can do to make sure the changes to your habits are permanent.

CHAPTER 8

DEVELOP GOOD EATING HABITS FOR RESULTS THAT LAST A LIFETIME

Okay. Now we know what to eat to make weight loss easy and keep hunger at bay. But we want to maintain this healthy eating for life. How? I learned that people who maintain their weight loss share a few very important habits that we can learn from. In addition, I discovered some neat tricks and tips of my own that will help keep your appetite under control and your weight steady.

KEEP A DAILY FOOD JOURNAL

Studies repeatedly have found that those who keep a log of their food intake have more consistent and successful weight loss and weight maintenance. I know this to be true from personal experience. I never kept a food journal until I began developing this plan. But when I did, it made a *big* difference.

I was surprised to find how easy it is to forget many of the foods you have eaten during the day, especially the bites of food you sneak in between meals. Yet they all add up. Remember, it takes only an extra 100 calories per day (a small slice of bread) to gain ten pounds in a year. An honest food journal will either prevent that from happening or at least show you where your extra weight is coming from while you think you're following a reasonable diet.

Keeping a food journal gave me an added bonus: I could track how each food affected me. I tracked how energetic or tired I felt after eating certain foods, and how satiated or quickly hungry I became again. So I learned which foods were more satisfying and which gave me energy boosts. I knew what snacks to avoid so I wouldn't feel fatigued. That's how I came to formulate my meal plans, and a journal will help you too.

A final caution: Make sure to measure your foods. Research shows that most people do not know how to measure portions. A portion is smaller than you think! A colleague once complained to me that she was gaining weight despite eating just 1,300 calories per day—500 fewer than her plan allowed. She admitted she was "eyeballing" her portions. Once she began measuring everything, she was shocked to learn she'd been eating closer to 3,000 calories per day. No wonder she was gaining weight!

WEIGH YOURSELF AT LEAST ONCE A WEEK

I never used to own a scale, and I was weighed only once a year at the doctor's office. But studies show that those who weigh themselves regularly tend to gain less weight and lose weight more consistently when cutting calories.

In fact, a 2006 study led by Rena Wing, PhD, at Brown University and the Miriam Hospital found the majority of research subjects who weighed in daily maintained their weight (within five pounds) more successfully than those who eschewed the scale.[7] Researchers attributed this to early awareness. In other words, if I'm getting on the scale regularly, I can spot an upward trend immediately and take action to curb it before I'm faced with ten extra pounds or more.

Weigh yourself naked first thing in the morning, after you've gone to the bathroom and before you've had anything to eat or drink. That's your absolute lowest weight, and you cannot fool yourself by shifting blame for any weight gain to your clothes. (Your jeans do not weigh ten pounds!)

Weight fluctuates, as you'll see when you get on the scale regularly. I never fully appreciated the effects of certain high-sodium foods on weight before. Now I see how temporary water retention gives me a little extra weight the day after a high-sodium nosh.

By keeping up this habit, you'll be able to track your weight trend—whether it's headed up or down—and take appropriate action.

HAVE A BEVERAGE WITH MEALS

Even though I'm not a big breakfast eater, I've always noticed that I am quickly satiated in the mornings. Whatever I eat, I enjoy it with a big cup of coffee. Apparently that's the key. My research taught me that drinking a hot beverage with a meal encourages faster satiation. Some studies suggest that people who drink hot or cold beverages with their meals tend to eat up to 20 percent fewer calories throughout the day than those who do not drink with meals.

I have definitely found this to be true, and many with whom I have shared this tip have told me this works for them too. I suspect it helps for two reasons. First, when you drink while you eat, it adds volume but few or no calories to your meal. (I drink tea, coffee with a little nondairy creamer, or some other no-calorie beverage like Crystal Light.) Second, I know for a fact that drinking with my meal causes me to eat more slowly, giving my brain a chance to signal that I am satiated before I have the chance to overeat.

---

7   See *New England Journal of Medicine*, October 12, 2006.

DRINK PLENTY OF WATER

We've all heard we should drink at least eight 8-ounce glasses of water each day—a rule I have been following for years. The research, however, is all over the place as to whether this is good or unnecessary. I read enough contradictory studies to test it myself.

I let my water intake drop to just a few glasses a day for about a week and a half. Not only did my weight go up dramatically—I went from my normal 107 to 108 pounds up to 113 pounds in *ten days*—but I noticed the creases in my forehead harshened noticeably. Plus, I was hungrier than usual. It turns out that water does a great job of keeping my appetite at bay.

I went back to my usual 64 ounces per day, and my weight went right back down to 108 in one week. The lines in my face lightened up. I know I didn't lose fat; my daily calorie intake and activity level didn't change, so I know that five-pound "loss" was really just loss of retained water weight.

I did some more research to find out why this might happen. Some studies indicate that while we may not need 64 ounces of water a day to be properly hydrated, the body does need a constant flow of water into the system to keep it from holding on to the water it has. In other words, when water is plentiful, there's no need for the body to hoard it.

We all have different needs. Eight glasses of water a day is more than enough for some of us. If you're extremely active, live in a hot, dry climate, or have certain medical conditions, you may need more water than the rest of us.

About eight glasses a day is perfect for me, and it works well for many people. Here's how I do it. I start my day with a 12-ounce glass of water as soon as I get out of bed. I'll admit, it's not easy to chug a big glass of water right away. But it hydrates you and starts to fill your stomach.

I drink the remaining water throughout the rest of the day. I always drink about 32 ounces with my workout. (I have a large canteen that works well for this.) I also drink one glass of water between meals. It really does help to knock out your appetite, and I think there's an added bonus for your skin.

Whenever I feel ravenously hungry, I always drink a glass of water (even if I've already had my 64 ounces) before I eat *anything*. Most of the time, it tempers the hunger enough that it puts me back in control and allows me to make intelligent choices about what I'm going to eat.

DON'T SKIP MEALS IN AN EFFORT TO SPEED WEIGHT LOSS

It may seem like a good idea to speed up your weight loss by skipping meals, but studies show that it always backfires. Slow and steady is the way to go for permanent results.

Remember, we're talking about a change from the lifestyle that caused you to reach an unacceptable weight. Opt for the lifestyle that will be satisfying and comfortable for your body and your mind. Skipping meals is just not a healthy way to live. And quite frankly, it sucks the enjoyment out of life. We should be able to enjoy our food and eat at regular intervals so we don't suffer that nasty, weak, shaky, famished feeling that comes from skipping meals.

Reducing calories beyond what is necessary for slow and steady weight loss is not helpful either. That kind of deprivation just screams "diet!" and a diet is something we go on to achieve a certain weight loss, then exit and return to our old habits. My plan should never feel like a diet—and it won't if you lose your excess weight in a slow, steady, and reasonable manner.

You want to be able to eat when you're legitimately hungry. I call it "legitimate hunger" when I haven't eaten in several hours and I feel hungry. And if I eat my 1,700 to 1,800 daily calorie allotment, I should be able to satisfy my legitimate hunger every day. I'm eating enough throughout the day that I rarely get that famished feeling that leads to overeating.

But if I were to shave off a couple hundred calories or start skipping meals to lose weight, I would follow some weak, famished mealtimes with a pig-out. I know, because I've done it. And medical research has shown this is true too. A study at the

University of Texas at Austin School of Nursing determined that the day before a binge, the women studied ate about 750 fewer calories than usual.[8] The researcher concluded that the feeling of deprivation likely triggered the binge. I try to avoid that now by not undereating.

TRY TO HAVE A
LATE-AFTERNOON SNACK

Sometimes I get hungry in the late afternoon, and that's when I like to eat my fruit. By this time of the day, I have already had two meals with adequate protein. Fruit, although very nutritious, is a carb, so I like to eat it either with a protein or in the hours following a meal that included protein.

Cherries, plums, apples, peaches, pears, and berries fall on the lower end of the glycemic index, as far as fruits go. I generally aim for a fruit with a GI rating of fifty-five or lower. That makes apples my typical afternoon snack. They're easy to carry with me, and I just love them. I have really gotten into enjoying the various types, from Rome apples, Jonathans, and Fujis to Red Delicious, Galas, and Cameos. Some are sweet, some are tart, and all have a fair amount of fiber.

As a bonus, a study found that subjects who ate an apple before a meal consumed 15 percent fewer calories during that meal.[9] The researchers attributed this to the fiber in the whole fruit, as the results were not the same with applesauce or apple juice.

You can have anything you want for your snack. I just like to eat my fruit completely by itself. If I eat fruit with other foods, especially vegetables, I get terribly bloated. Not fun. That's why my late-afternoon snack is a great time to have it.

Occasionally I'll swap my fruit for some tea and veggies with dip or cucumber spears sprinkled with lemon pepper. Other times, I'll have some dry-roasted almonds. Once in a while, we all have one of those days where we just feel hungry all day. That's

---

8   Study conducted by Gayle M. Timmerman, University of Texas at Austin School of Nursing, 1998.
9   Study conducted by Barbara J. Rolls, Pennsylvania State University, 2007.

when I'll opt for some straight protein, like string cheese or a few rolled-up pieces of turkey or lean ham.

It really doesn't matter what you eat (although I wouldn't recommend a starchy treat—you don't want to tank your blood sugar and trigger your appetite) as long as you stay within your snack calorie allotment.

HAVE A PIG-OUT MEAL ONCE A WEEK

Schedule one pig-out meal every week. At this meal, you can splurge a bit—within reason—without worrying that you have blown it.

This weekly pig-out is part of the plan, so once you've stayed within your daily calorie allotment all week, you get this treat.

Many experts now agree that such planned splurges, as long as they're reasonable, go a long way toward helping us to maintain better eating habits the majority of the time. Why? They prevent us from feeling deprived, a prime culprit of bingeing. I know it works for me.

But don't go hog wild and eat everything in sight. For pig-outs, just enjoy a meal or dessert within reason, without focusing on the carb/protein/fat ratio and the calories. Simply enjoy the food.

When I say "within reason," I mean the pig-out meal is not a green light to take in all the calories you just reduced all week. That's self-defeating. Just try to be rational and sensible about it. Don't have two cheeseburgers and fries, but you can have one. Don't have two milk shakes. Have just one. Don't eat the whole carton of ice cream, but you can have a good-sized bowl.

Having said that, I'll tell you there have been many times when my pig-out proceeded from a reasonable treat of 500 or 600 extra calories to well over 1,000. And now I know why. Studies show that whenever we blend a multitude of tastes (sweet, salty, sour, etc.) and textures (creamy, crunchy, chewy . . .), we eat more. (see Chapter Seven, Don't Eat Too Much Variety.) So now, I determine exactly what it is I am

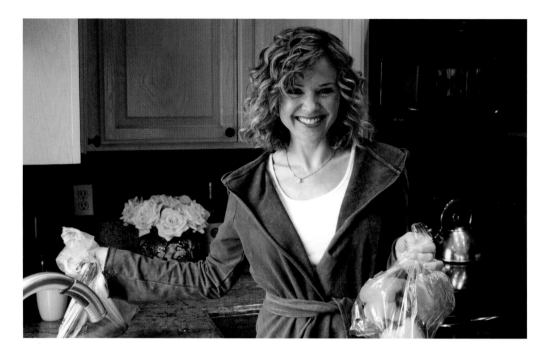

craving, and I try to eat just that. Resist jumping from chocolate to ice cream to chips to cookies. You'll eat less in your pig-outs when you choose just one thing and stick to it.

I don't worry about the extra 500 or 600 pig-out calories. But on those occasions where I've gone too far and eaten 1,000 extra calories or more, I'll do about thirty extra minutes of cardio the next day and cut back a bit on my calories.

I've always found it helpful to know that I could have that pig-out meal every week, especially in the early years of developing my plan. It made it much easier to ignore the temptation of my favorite high-calorie foods every day, knowing there was a set time when I could indulge a bit without derailing my whole eating plan.

It's like getting your paycheck and paying your bills first, but setting some aside for later. You enjoy that shopping spree or movie night so much more when you know you've taken care of business by paying your bills and meeting your obligations first. Now you've earned your fun!

So decide exactly what you're craving, and plan to have that for your pig-out. Don't eat around it—go for the gold.

By the way, if I'm really craving a crazy, high-calorie dessert, like one of those chocolate lava cakes at my favorite restaurants, I'll very occasionally trade my traditional healthy dinner for a piece of cake with a cup of coffee. Mmmm! I know this is nutritionally horrible, but it doesn't kill me to do it once in a great while. And it has kept me on the straight and narrow throughout many weeks, knowing I could do something ridiculous like that without completely blowing my progress.

RESTAURANT RULES

Restaurant meals are not the enemies you might think they are. You have to be prepared, and you need to ask for a few minor adjustments, but you can eat out and still lose weight. I have found that almost all restaurants are more than willing to help. Here's how I approach eating out.

1. If you can, do a little Internet research before you visit the restaurant. See what nutrition information you can dig up on the menu items when you go. I almost always do this, and it gives me a few ideas for what to order before I get there. You can start with the restaurant's Web site, or type the restaurant's name into your favorite search engine. The legwork is especially valuable when you arrive famished. It's nearly impossible not to order the most fattening foods once you're hungry—unless you have arrived with a plan.

2. As soon as you sit down, drink a glass of water. It will begin to fill your stomach and allow you to make your selections without being quite as hungry.

3. Order a hot beverage, or at least a low- or no-calorie beverage, to have with your meal. Wine and other alcoholic beverages count as carbs, or starch. If you order one, skip the starch with your meal. Substitute a low-glycemic vegetable (like broccoli, bell peppers, zucchini, cauliflower, or green beans) for the bread, potato, rice, corn, or peas.

4. Whenever possible, order a green salad with dressing on the side (and no croutons, bacon bits, egg, or cheese) to begin your meal. If there are no good

selections of side salads to choose from, I will ask for a side of steamed broccoli, or any other low-glycemic veggie (such as zucchini, asparagus, bell peppers, or cauliflower) as an appetizer. Along with the beverage, this will start to fill you up with low-calorie, high-volume foods so you're less likely to overeat during the rest of the meal.

5. Share a meal if you can. I almost always do unless I want fish, which no one else in my family usually wants. If I'm not sharing a meal, I ask for a "to go" box before the meal is even served. I put half the food in there as soon as it arrives. Out of sight, out of mind. Besides, I always look forward to enjoying the leftovers (with a big salad or Holly's Roasted Veggies) as one of my meals the next day. Another option is to order an appetizer as your main course. The portion is smaller, so you'll be less likely to overeat.

6. Order low-glycemic vegetables as your side dish with your main meal. Ask for them steamed or roasted with only a little bit of oil or butter. Or ask for them prepared with no oil, then get some butter on the side so you can control how much you use.

    Broccoli is my go-to veggie, whether I'm cooking at home or eating out. Not only is broccoli low-glycemic, high in fiber, and filled with antioxidants, it has the added bonus of protein—2.6 grams of protein (and just thirty-one calories) in a one-cup serving. Even if it's not listed on the menu, most restaurants are happy to bring you an order of steamed broccoli with butter on the side.

7. Try to order the simplest foods on the menu. Choose from baked, broiled, grilled, poached, roasted, stir-fried, or steamed entrées with the fewest sauces and other extras. Ask that your meal be cooked with no extra salt, butter, or oil. Steer clear of fried, crispy, and creamed dishes at all costs. They're just high-calorie disasters. Also avoid stuffed, buttered, and breaded foods.

    I try to order grilled chicken or broiled fish rather than, say, chicken cordon bleu or fried fish served in cream sauce. If there are no simple dishes on the menu, order all sauces, gravies, creams, and oils on the side. That way you can add just a little for flavor without loading up on extra calories.

If you can't stand it, and you simply have to order a rich, creamy dish, either split it with someone else or make sure to put half in a to-go box immediately. Be extra careful to really fill up on your salad and veggies first so you don't overeat the calorie-rich entrée. Think of it more as a dessert rather than as part of your meal.

8. You can have unlimited low-glycemic veggies and salad (with butter, oils, and dressing on the side). Beyond that, use these guidelines:

   - Half of your fist—that's your starch or carb portion

   - The palm of your hand—that's your lean protein portion

   - Stick out your thumb—that's the portion for fat, including cheese. (Make sure to cut off all visible fat, as there can be a lot of hidden fats in restaurant foods. Remove the skin from chicken, and cut away visible fat from a steak.)

9. As a visual aid, half your plate is filled with salad and non-starchy veggies. The other half of the plate is divided in two quarters. One quarter is your lean protein, and the other is your starch or carb portion.

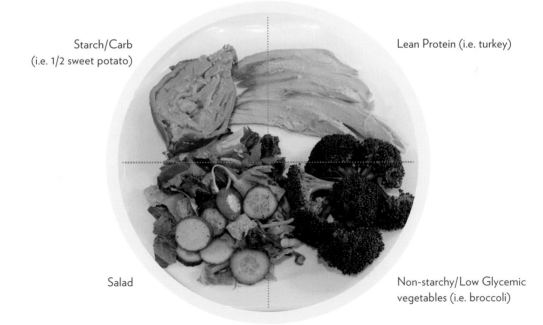

Starch/Carb (i.e. 1/2 sweet potato)

Lean Protein (i.e. turkey)

Salad

Non-starchy/Low Glycemic vegetables (i.e. broccoli)

10. If you order a sandwich or hamburger, remove one of the slices of bread. (I peel away the top layer of bread as I eat the sandwich, so I have something to hold on to when I'm eating. But I've skipped eating an entire piece of bread by the time I've finished. I never miss it.)

11. Order sandwiches and burgers "dry"—no oils like mayonnaise and special sauces. Use as much mustard as you want or a little bit of ketchup (ketchup is fairly high in sugar, so be judicious).

12. Sour cream and guacamole add a couple hundred extra calories to a burrito, so either order them on the side or do what I do and replace them with salsa.

13. For restaurant breakfasts, order eggs à la carte with a carb on the side—dry wheat toast, half a dry bagel, or a small serving of oatmeal. Poached eggs are the most waistline-friendly, since there's no oil or butter added. But I prefer mine scrambled, so I don't worry about the oil used to scramble the eggs as long as what I'm eating them with is dry.

KICK-START YOUR WEIGHT LOSS!

All right. You already have my stress-reduction tools. I have now given you all the tricks and all my secrets to eating right so you will *enjoy* your weight loss. In Part III, I'll show you how I exercise to get the best results with maximum efficiency. (We aren't going to be spending hours at the gym!) But let me also give you something personal. In Chapter Eleven, I have listed an entire month of exactly what I ate, exactly what I did for exercise, and most important, what I did each morning to set myself up for a low-stress, successful day. I have done this to make it as easy as possible for you to follow along and make this plan your own. Feel free to make a photocopy of Chapter Eleven and keep it with you. Take it with you when you grocery shop, when you work out, and to help you tackle stress during your day. Many people have told me they love that they can simply follow exactly what I do so there is no guesswork, no thinking, just ahhhhh.

PART THREE

REVAMP
THE WAY
YOU'RE
EXERCISING

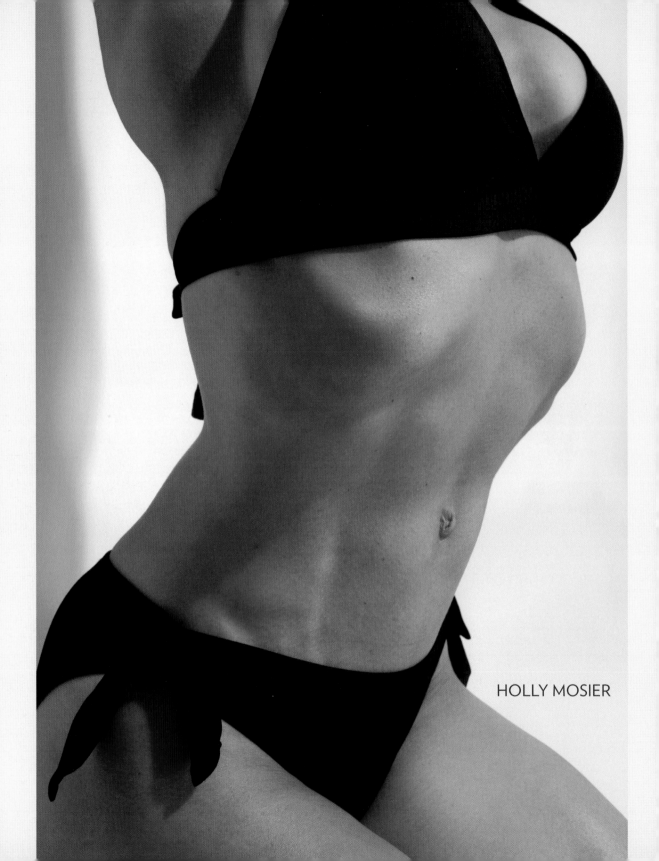

HOLLY MOSIER

CHAPTER 9

HOLLY'S GUIDELINES FOR OPTIMAL EXERCISE

For decades, I exercised for about ninety minutes nearly every day. It worked, too . . . until I hit my forties and the weight started to inch up anyway. Adding more time to my daily workout just wasn't an option. Besides, I was also dealing with fatigue. It was all I could do to get those ninety minutes in!

What a relief to discover it wasn't necessary. My research revealed that I could make my workouts more efficient and get better results with just one hour of exercise per day and maybe one day off each week. It has worked beautifully for me for years now, and I'll share those secrets with you in this chapter.

Some days I'll exceed an hour—like on the days I do half an hour of cardio as well as a yoga class. But other days I do a lot less—about thirty minutes of just cardio. It averages out to about an hour a day. That's what most recent studies on weight control say you should aim for, and I agree with them.

I still follow all those corny little suggestions to incorporate extra activity into my day. I'm one of those people who parks way out in a parking lot and walks in. I usually take the stairs rather than an elevator, and I try to walk my dog every day. That's about fifteen minutes. I look for every opportunity to move.

GUIDELINE ONE: EXERCISE EVERY DAY FOR ABOUT FORTY-FIVE TO SIXTY MINUTES

There's just no way around this. You've probably heard the standard recommendation to work out at least three days per week, but I find that three or four days a week just doesn't cut it if you want steady and permanent weight loss. And studies on obesity are finding this is true. Those who have the best long-term results are those who exercise a *minimum* of five days per week.

For years, many scientific studies advised at least thirty minutes of moderate exercise five days per week for weight loss, but the experts are beginning to change their tune. That amount of exercise offers a multitude of health benefits, including improved mood and reduced risk for many chronic diseases, such as coronary heart disease and diabetes, but it's not adequate for permanent weight loss.

The American College of Sports Medicine (ACSM) now says it's necessary to exercise at least forty-five to sixty minutes most days of the week to lose weight and maintain that weight loss. And I have certainly found that is true.

I tested various workout lengths and frequencies as I developed my plan, closely monitoring the results of my ninety-minute daily workouts for several weeks. I also tried the thirty-minute sessions five days a week to see if I could get by with that. (The answer: not by a long shot.)

If you want to lose weight and keep it off, you have to commit to an hour of exercise a day, most days. With that said, you do not have to have killer workouts every day. Not at all. The ACSM says "moderate-intensity" exercise at least three hundred minutes per week will do the job. Not surprisingly, the ACSM also states that more exercise of higher intensity will bring greater weight-loss and maintenance results.

So how do you know if yours is a "moderate-intensity" workout or a "high-intensity" routine? Examples of moderate-intensity exercise include exerting light effort on a stationary bike or cycling outdoors for leisure, not at racing speeds. Higher-intensity activities include jogging, calisthenics, and faster running—basically, anything that gets your heart really pumping and causes you to be out of breath at times.

For the greatest efficiency and consistent results, I generally blend these two intensities in my workouts. I'll explain the specifics later (in guideline six), but I want to assure you up front that you do not need forty-five to sixty minutes of constant high-intensity exercise to lose weight and maintain it.

You don't even have to do your forty-five to sixty minutes all at one time during the day. If you're too busy to carve out that much time at once, break it into smaller segments throughout the day. Studies have found that three ten-minute sessions are just as effective as one thirty-minute workout, and I have found this to be true.

GUIDELINE TWO: VARY YOUR ACTIVITIES AND WORKOUTS

No doubt we are more consistent exercisers when we do things we like to do—and consistency delivers results. You may believe you have to do certain types of exercise to lose weight and maintain it, but it's the rare person who can dredge up the willpower to hammer out a workout he or she hates doing, day after day.

Instead, have lots of different activities and workouts to choose from. You don't have to limit your exercise to cardio and weights at the gym or a group exercise class. Anything that gets your heart pumping counts. My aim is to at least break a mild sweat every day, and I can do that while I'm walking my dog.

Mixing up your exercise (sometimes called cross-training) helps enormously in resculpting your body and avoiding injury. For many years, I performed the same ninety-minute routine. I started on the stationary bike with a forty-five-minute, moderate-intensity ride. Next, I proceeded to the same weight-lifting routine every single day. I did grow very strong—at one point, I could nearly bench-press my weight! But I never achieved the lean, sinewy look I was after. And later, the same static workout pattern proved ineffective for weight loss and maintenance. After I turned forty, checking in daily at the gym to grind out the same old program wasn't enough to prevent a one- or two-pound gain each year.

Choose the activities you like the most (or hate the least), and you'll be less likely to wimp out on getting your sixty minutes of daily exercise. Tennis, racquetball, hiking, swimming, surfing, kayaking, cycling, walking (especially in hilly areas), gardening, skating, waterskiing, snow skiing, boxing, yoga, Pilates, tai chi, tae kwon do, and dancing (even at a nightclub, it counts as exercise!) are all moderate- to high-intensity activities. Pick up a game of basketball or soccer; play baseball with the kids or go for a bike ride. Mow the lawn. Climb steps at the beach, or take your table tennis game with you. Join a volleyball league. Take a spin class or any of the plethora of group exercise classes offered at the gym or YMCA. Do different things every day or every week. It's all good, and it all counts.

Studies have confirmed that the more fun you have while exercising, the less you'll feel like you exerted yourself. In other words, you won't be as exhausted from a fun game of beach volleyball as you might if you had planted yourself on a stationary bike for the same amount of time. And if you perceive your exercise as fun, you'll want to do it—and do it regularly.

GUIDELINE THREE: DO CARDIO EXERCISE AND RESISTANCE TRAINING

Back in the '80s and '90s, cardio exercise was considered much more important than resistance training for weight loss and maintenance. In fact, it was common throughout those decades for people to perform cardio almost exclusively, like riding a stationary bike or taking an aerobics class.

Today we know that resistance training plays a huge role in weight control. Muscles atrophy as we get older, and because muscle burns up to seven times more calories at rest than fat does, that also causes our metabolism to plummet. If your body has more fat and less muscle than it did ten years ago, that means you'll gain weight eating the same number of calories you used to because your metabolism has slowed.

So of course it follows that the greater your muscle mass, the higher your metabolism. Resistance training builds muscle, boosting metabolism.

Although cardio burns a lot of calories and strengthens your heart and lungs, you need resistance training to prevent the muscle atrophy that occurs with age. Cardio alone doesn't do much to sculpt your body, especially your upper body. Resistance training helps you tone and shape the muscles.

Weight lifting is one form of resistance training, but it's not your only choice. Anything that uses your body weight will do. Push-ups are a classic example. Yoga and Pilates both utilize resistance training. Resistance bands (those long, stretchy tubes with handles on each end) are another great option; plus, they're easy to pack for traveling.

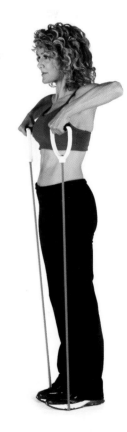

I particularly like activities that combine cardio and resistance, like boxing. You get a great cardio workout, but you also get resistance training when you hit the bag. Swimming combines cardio and resistance as you push against the water. Martial arts also combine the two as you punch or kick against a bag or an opponent.

If you choose weights for your resistance training, you should take a day or two off in between weight sessions. Your muscles need time to recuperate. Daily resistance training of this sort strains the muscles and joints and sets you up for injuries.

And although there may be some who disagree with me, I don't think doing yoga every day is good, either. When I was doing yoga almost daily through my months of yoga teacher training, I came away from it with a very sore left shoulder and what is comically referred to as "yoga butt," a chronic inflammation at the top of the hamstring where it attaches to the sit bone. Those injuries took several months to heal.

This is why I am a fan of varying activities and workouts. I rarely do the same exercise routine or activity two days in a row. (In Chapter Eleven, I give you a month's worth of my actual workouts so you can see how I vary this.) Constantly mixing it up continues to challenge your muscles in new and different ways, and that results in a more well-rounded physique and fewer injuries.

GUIDELINE FOUR: AIM TO BURN AT LEAST 250 TO 350 CALORIES PER DAY WITH EXERCISE

Guidelines vary as to how many calories per day we should aim to burn with exercise. Some recommend burning at least 200 per day; others preach that we must burn much more to lose weight and maintain it.

According to the most recent ACSM guidelines, you need to exercise two hundred to three hundred minutes per week and burn 2,000 calories in order to lose or maintain weight. If you exercise six days a week, that comes out to forty-five to sixty minutes of exercise per day and about 325 calories per session.

In a 2008 *Prevention* magazine article, Oprah Winfrey's trainer, Bob Greene, recommended exercising five or six times per week, burning 200 to 300 calories per session. I used the suggestion and found that it worked to maintain my weight at about 107 pounds if I ate my regular 1,700 to 1,800 calories per day. Some days I burn a little less than 200 calories (like when I'm doing only thirty minutes of cardio and don't push too hard); others, I burn well over 300 (whenever I take a boxing class).

But I believe all your activity counts. So even if you burn only 200 calories in your exercise session, if you continue to move during the day—walking your kids to school, taking the stairs rather than the elevator—you'll probably get closer to that 300-calorie mark than you'd think. But you have to keep moving throughout the day, not just during your "official" exercise session.

Be aware that we all burn calories at different rates. Larger people burn more calories than smaller people. A large man will burn a lot more calories than a small woman while doing the same activity. My husband burns about 650 calories in the same boxing class where I burn 325.

In fact, when you see those charts that state how many calories a person burns while doing a specific activity (like "an hour of jogging burns 476 calories"), they are almost always based on an "average-sized" person. That is usually a 150-pound person. You'll burn more or less, depending on your size, your age, and your metabolism.

How many calories are you burning? That brings us to guideline five.

Get the right tools and you'll know.

GUIDELINE FIVE: USE A HEART-RATE MONITOR FOR THE MOST EFFICIENT EXERCISE

You can actually exercise less if you do it more efficiently. Start by educating yourself about your target heart rate range and making sure that you're falling into that range when you exercise. The easiest way to do this is by wearing a heart-rate monitor.

There are many different types and models. Some are simple and others are quite complex. The best are those that display your heart rate and how many calories you've burned. These help you ensure you're exercising at the proper intensity and hitting your target for calories burned—the epitome of exercising efficiently.

Thanks to this handy tool, I now know why I was getting poorer results with longer workouts. During my old ninety-minute sessions, I was working far below my target heart rate and burning fewer calories than I do now with shorter workouts.

I don't make that mistake now. I almost always wear a heart-rate monitor during my exercise so I know when I need to exert more effort and when I can back off a bit. That has allowed me to reduce my cardio from at least forty-five minutes per day to around thirty, with much better results. My monitor also calculates how many calories I've burned, making my exercise sessions wickedly efficient.

WHAT'S MY TARGET HEART RATE?

What is your target heart rate? It varies according to your age and fitness level.

I have made it easy for you with a simple calculator at www.hollymosier.com. If you don't have access to a computer, you can use this general formula: Subtract your age from 220. Multiply that number by 60 percent to determine the bottom number in your target heart-rate range. Next, multiply that number by 80 percent to determine the highest number in your range.

For example, for a forty-year-old with an average fitness level, the 60 percent formula would look like this: $220 - 40 = 180 \times .60 = 108$ beats per minute. The 80 percent formula would look like this: $220 - 40 = 180 \times .80 = 144$ beats per minute. The target heart-rate range is 108 to 144. That person should maintain a heart rate in this range throughout the cardio workout.

The formula changes a bit for those who are very fit. These are people who have been exercising consistently and vigorously for quite a while. For them, the range is 70 percent to 90 percent. So for a forty-year-old who is superfit, the 70 percent formula would look like this: $220 - 40 = 180 \times .70 = 126$. The 90 percent formula would look like this: $220 - 40 = 180 \times .90 = 162$. The target heart-rate zone is 126 to 162 beats per minute. That person should aim for this zone while doing cardio.

Another great way to learn your target heart-rate range is to be assessed by a knowledgeable personal trainer. A good trainer will take all these factors into account and monitor you during your exercise sessions to ensure you're working in the proper range for your age and fitness level. If I were just starting out, I would definitely invest in this. It would have saved me years of exercising inefficiently and achieving less than optimal results.

HOW HARD DO I HAVE TO EXERCISE?

Within that broad target heart-rate range, where should you aim to spend most of that cardio session? That depends on your fitness level. Beginners should start with the 60 percent formula. As you get more fit, move up from there. For those of average fitness, reach for the higher 80 percent target for part of your cardio session. If you're already very fit, go for the 90 percent target for some of your cardio session.

Whatever your fitness level, work at the top end of your target heart-rate range for only about 20 percent of your workout. For 80 percent of your workout, you should keep to the middle or low end of your target heart-rate range to help you avoid overtraining and burnout. How do you do that? Easy. It's called "interval training," and I address that next.

GUIDELINE SIX:
USE INTERVAL TRAINING

The key to reducing the time you work out, while still getting better results, is interval training. What is interval training? Interval training is where you exercise at a moderate pace punctuated with short bursts of high-intensity effort. So interval training dictates that rather than exercising at a steady pace, you work primarily at the lower to middle end of your target heart-rate range, punctuated by short bursts of greater intensity that drive your heart rate up to the upper limits of your range for a brief period. When you return to the slower pace, your heart rate slowly comes back down. Then you repeat the pattern, alternating between moderate- and high-intensity exercise.

Studies have found interval training is the most time-effective way to exercise for weight loss. A 2006 study noted that a thirty-minute cardio workout with intervals of four minutes of moderate cardio activity alternating with thirty-second bursts of high-intensity cardio activity is essentially as effective as ninety minutes of cardio at a consistent and moderate heart rate.[10] I have experimented with many varieties of intervals (for example, three minutes of moderate cardio alternated with three minutes of high intensity) and found them all to be very effective. But here's the pattern I have found works like magic for me.

I begin my cardio—whether on the stationary bike, elliptical machine, treadmill, or even jogging—with a three-minute warm-up. At minute three, I begin my first interval

---

10   Gibala, M.J., Jonathan P. Little, Martin van Essen, et al., "Short-Term Sprint Interval versus Traditional Endurance Training," *Journal of Physiology* 575, September 15, 2006, 901–911.

by increasing my effort for thirty seconds, then returning to the more moderate pace until minute six. At minute six, I increase the intensity for thirty seconds again, then return to the moderate pace. At minute nine, I increase the pace for a full minute, then return to the moderate pace. At minute 12:30, I do another thirty-second burst. At minute fifteen, I do another one. Then another at minute eighteen, and a final thirty-second burst at 20:30 or 21:00. That makes for a total of seven intervals.

After I complete my final interval, I just continue on with my moderate pace until I've burned about 200 calories, which usually comes between minute thirty and minute thirty-three, depending on how hard I've worked during the session.

I experimented with many, many patterns before settling on this one, which seems to fit my body and fitness level very well. You can and should experiment with a wide variety of interval patterns. Find the ones that challenge you, feel good, and are enjoyable to do. I started with a pattern of four minutes of moderate intensity followed by thirty seconds of higher intensity, but I wasn't burning 200 calories in thirty minutes. I increased the intensity of the pattern a bit to match my goal.

A final suggestion: Sync your music on your iPod to match the intervals you choose. You'll feel like a rock star.

GUIDELINE SEVEN:
DO NOT OVERTRAIN

There's a pervasive belief in our culture that if a little of something is good, more must be better. Not true. Too much of anything is always counterproductive. You can even drink too much water. It is the balance of activity and rest that results in good health and increased energy.

So, what is overtraining? It's when you've engaged in too much activity and exercise without enough rest to counterbalance it. It can also occur if you exercise at too high an intensity for much of your exercise sessions. What constitutes "too much" varies greatly from person to person, but there are common indicators to watch for.

Not surprisingly, one of the most prevalent symptoms of overtraining is lethargy and fatigue. It can also cause increased or decreased appetite, sleep disruption, and increase in frequency of colds, flu, and other illnesses as the body becomes more depleted. Muscle and joint soreness doesn't go away. If you don't back off when your body starts to signal it's time to do so, injuries become a lot more likely.

One excellent way to avoid overtraining is to always vary your activities (see guideline two) so you are constantly working different muscles and muscle groups rather than targeting the same muscles every day. That gives the muscles some time to rest.

Another way is to wear your heart-rate monitor to ensure that when you work out, you're working in your target heart-rate zone and not above it. Plus, the heart-rate monitor will allow you to balance your effort so you are not working at the top end of your target heart-rate zone for more than 20 percent of your workout.

And you need adequate rest, including plenty of sleep. This means not only backing off the exercise when you're injured or sick, but also getting ample sleep every night. Studies have found that when athletes received less than optimal sleep, their athletic performance suffered.

Listen to your body. It will let you know if you're overdoing it. There's nothing wrong with taking a few days off if you need to. Take two or three days and just walk those days, laying off everything else. You'll be refreshed when you go back to more vigorous activity. The only caution: If you take a break from exercise for more than a day or two, make sure to reduce your daily calorie allotment to compensate for the calories you are not burning through your regular exercise sessions.

GUIDELINE EIGHT:
HAVE A CUP OF COFFEE TO BOOST YOUR WORKOUTS

I love coffee. Just the smell of it brewing makes me happy. Coffee was always my dad's beverage of choice, and I grew up in a household that embraced it. So I have been particularly pleased about the most recent studies finding that coffee has a multitude of health and fitness benefits for those who have no medical reasons not to imbibe.

(Note: Consult your doctor before beginning any nutrition and exercise program. Certain physical conditions and illnesses can be exacerbated by drinking coffee. Please consult medical professionals before following any suggestions here, to ensure you can safely practice them.)

I like to drink a small but strong cup of fresh-brewed coffee about thirty minutes before my workout. It's the caffeine in the coffee that makes working out seem easier. According to a 2005 British review of twenty-one different studies, caffeine not only decreased subjects' perceived rate of exertion during their exercise session by 5.6 percent, it also enhanced their performance by 11 percent.[11] I certainly feel like it helps me. What's more, coffee is loaded with antioxidants. Antioxidants help rid the body of free radicals, those pesky molecules that damage our cells and DNA, causing myriad nasties, from cancer and heart disease to strokes and wrinkles. In fact, studies have found coffee is America's main source of antioxidants, as we typically do not eat enough fruits and vegetables.

Studies also have linked coffee consumption to a lower risk of type 2 (insulin-resistant) diabetes and certain cancers. Other studies have found it may reduce the risk of dementia later in life and possibly delay Alzheimer's disease. Still more research suggests that coffee consumption could reduce the risk of Parkinson's disease. So in addition to being an exercise booster, coffee may offer many other health benefits. That's why it's my caffeine beverage of choice.

If you don't like coffee, you can still get the exercise boost and many of the same health benefits (as well as some others) from tea—especially green tea and black tea.

GUIDELINE NINE: CALENDAR YOUR DAILY WORKOUTS

As a final guideline, I have found it immensely helpful to schedule my daily workouts in my calendar as I would any other important appointment.

---

11 Doherty, M., and P.M. Smith, "Effects of Caffeine Ingestion on Rating of Perceived Exertion During and After Exercise," *Scandinavian Journal of Medicine & Science in Sports*, Volume 15 (2), April 2005, 69–78.

I usually put together my workout schedule for the week on Sunday night. If I have to miss an exercise session for any reason, I immediately get out the calendar and reschedule it. That way, I rarely miss. And it is this consistency that brings the results.

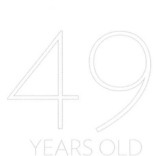

49
YEARS OLD

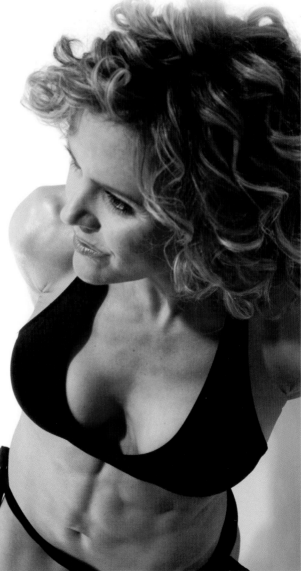

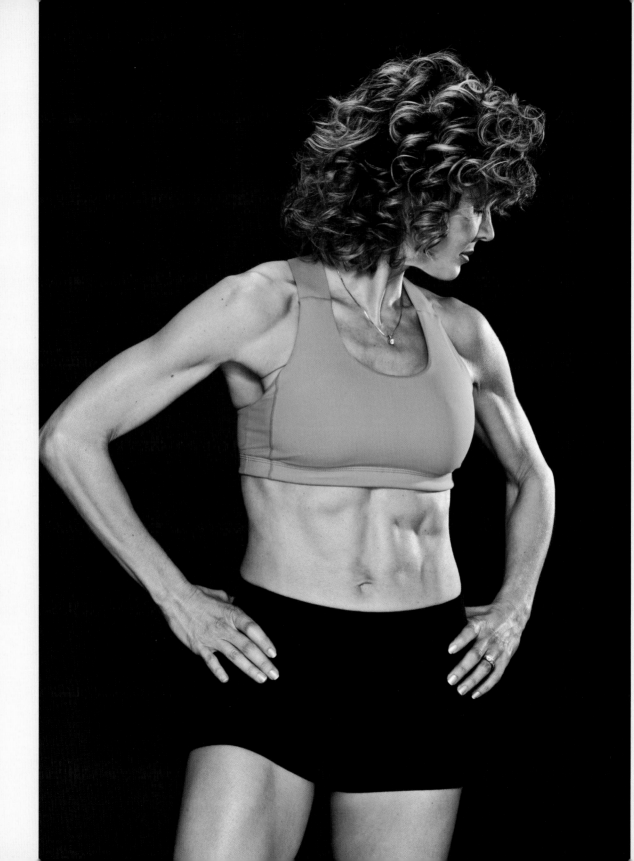

CHAPTER 10

HOLLY'S WORKOUT ROUTINES

I love being active, and I love being in shape, but I don't love living at the gym. I figured out the most efficient and effective workout routines so it will just look like you spend hours every day at the gym. That's what I was after.

In this chapter I am going to give you what I actually do for my gym workouts (cardio and weights), my go-to ab exercises for creating a sexy stomach, and my favorite group exercise classes. Then I will give you a quick and easy thirty-five-minute at-home boxing routine to do if you are time-crunched. And finally, in Chapter Eleven, I will give you thirty-one days of my actual workouts to show you how I put it all together.

Before we get to the workouts, I want to again emphasize the importance of interval training and a variety of activities. My results vastly improved when I gave up my static ninety-minute workout and embraced interval training and a wider variety of activities. Now I change up my exercise routine all the time. Some days I go to the gym for cardio and a light weight workout. Some days I take a group exercise class. Other days I go for a hike or stay home and jump rope or jog.

One day a week (and occasionally two), I only walk. On my walking day, I usually do about four miles. Many times I'll break this up and walk two miles in the morning and two miles later in the day. It's just as effective. And I usually either take two yoga classes per week, or, if it's a busy week and I can't fit two formal classes in, I'll do my Ten-Minute Yoga Sequences. On the days I do yoga, I usually do about twenty-five to thirty minutes of cardio.

As you can see, it's a lot of variety, and I switch it up all the time. Not only does this variety keep my workouts fresh but, it also requires my body to respond to different routines, which maximizes my fitness.

And finally, consistency in exercising is most important. You want to move your body for forty-five minutes to an hour every day, whether that is done by walking or a more formal exercise session. But please, don't beat yourself up or feel like you've failed if you don't do a formal exercise session that day. Just get out there and move!

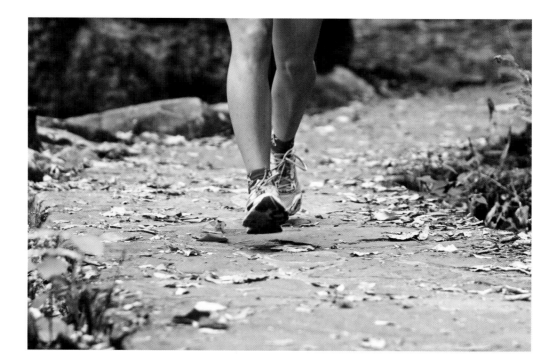

HOLLY'S **GYM WORKOUT**

When I do a regular gym-type workout, I usually start with cardio, then light weights, followed by ab exercises and stretching. Here is the routine that works best for me, and I know it will work for you.

1. Thirty minutes of cardio, using interval training techniques

2. Fifteen minutes of light weights

3. Three to five minutes of abdominal exercises

4. Five to ten minutes of stretching/yoga, sometimes including one of my Ten-Minute Yoga Sequences

1. THIRTY MINUTES OF **CARDIO**

I choose a different cardio exercise almost every day. Some days I'll ride the stationary bike; others I'll hop on the elliptical machine. Maybe I'll split my time between the bike, elliptical, and treadmill or finish up with five minutes on the rowing machine. I also love the VersaClimber, a machine that replicates climbing a ladder. I'll use any piece of cardio equipment the gym has! The only rule is to not use the same one all the time. Mix it up! If you use the stationary bike one day, pick a different cardio machine the next. Variety is the spice of life and the key to a well-rounded physique.

And remember, no matter what piece of cardio equipment you use, make sure to do interval cardio. Vary your heart rate for the best results.

2. FIFTEEN MINUTES OF LIGHT WEIGHTS

When I use weights, I do full-body weight training with *very* light weights (usually three to five pounds if I am using hand weights and about twenty pounds of resistance if I am using the exercise machines). I perform twelve to twenty repetitions and three sets per body area.

To work out my chest, I do one or two sets of **CHEST PRESSES**, then one or two sets of **CHEST FLIES**.

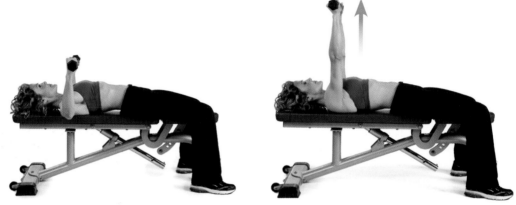

CHEST PRESSES: Lie back on a bench with your feet on the floor, holding your hand weights. Bring your arms to a T position, with your elbows bent at ninety-degree angles and your palms facing away from you. Press your arms straight up, then lower them back down.

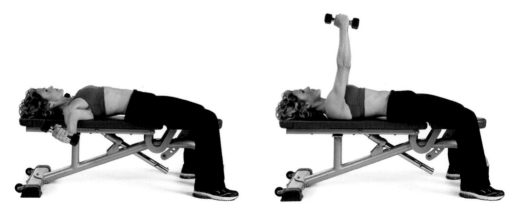

CHEST FLIES: Lie back on a bench with your feet on the floor, holding your hand weights. Open your arms to each side with your elbows slightly bent and your palms facing in. Bring your palms together over your chest, then lower your arms back down.

For my back, I do one or two sets of **DUMBBELL ROWS**, then one or two sets of **REVERSE FLIES**.

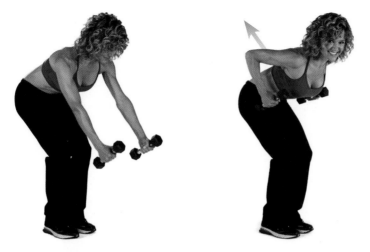

DUMBBELL ROWS: Stand with your feet hip-width apart, holding your hand weights. Slightly bend your knees and lean forward until your torso is at about a forty-five-degree angle. Extend your arms in front of you. Then perform a "rowing" motion by drawing your elbows back to your torso. Extend your arms out in front of you to return to the starting position.

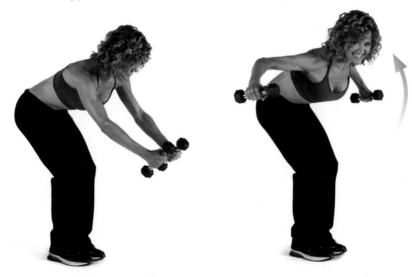

REVERSE FLIES: Stand with your feet hip-width apart, holding your hand weights. Slightly bend your knees and lean forward until your torso is at about a forty-five-degree angle. Extend your arms in front of you with your palms facing in. Keeping your elbows slightly bent, open your arms to either side, squeezing the shoulder blades together. Lower your arms back to the starting position.

For shoulders, I do a set or two of **SHOULDER FLIES**, then one or two sets of **OVERHEAD PRESSES**.

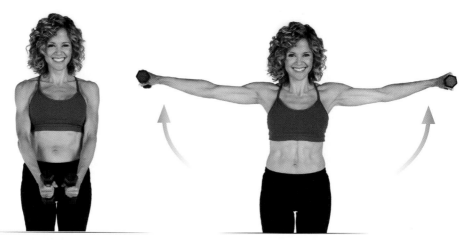

SHOULDER FLIES: Stand with your feet hip-width apart, holding your hand weights. With your arms extended down, bring your hands together in front of you with your palms facing in. Keep your elbows slightly bent and lift your arms up to either side, no higher than shoulder level. Lower your arms back down to the starting position.

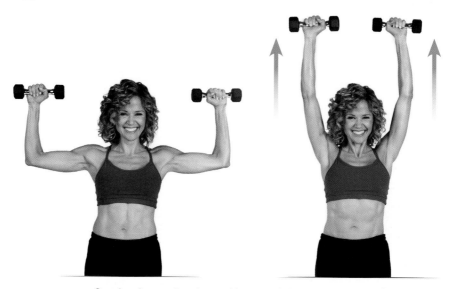

OVERHEAD PRESSES: Stand with your feet hip-width apart, holding your hand weights. Lift your arms to shoulder height and bend your elbows to ninety-degree angles with your palms facing forward. Press your arms straight up, then lower them back down to the starting position.

For my arms, I do about three sets for triceps (usually **TRICEPS DIPS**), and a set or two for biceps (usually **BICEPS CURLS**).

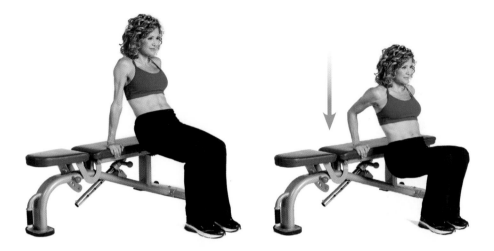

TRICEPS DIPS: Sit on the edge of a bench (or chair). Hold on to the edge with your hands, with your knees bent and your feet flat on the floor. Straighten your arms and slide off the bench. Bend your elbows to "dip" your hips, then press back up. (Do not bend your elbows more than ninety degrees.)

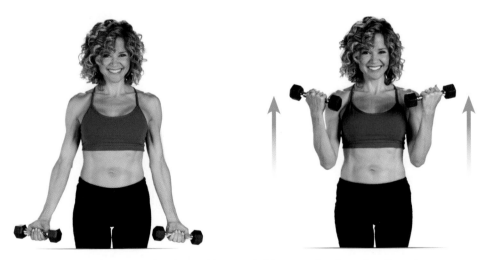

BICEPS CURLS: Stand with your feet hip-width apart, holding your hand weights. Extend your arms straight down, palms facing forward, leaving a slight bend at the elbows. Bend your arms, "curling" the weights to your chest, then lower your arms back down.

I'll sometimes add about three sets of **LUNGES** for my butt.

I finish with three to four minutes of concentrated abdominal work (which I explain on the following pages in its own section).

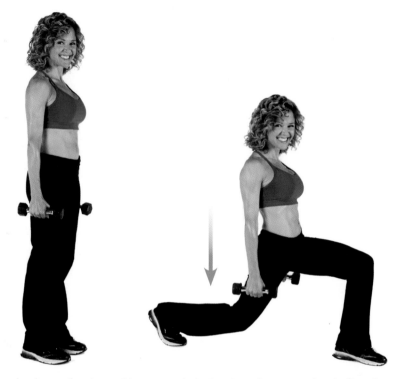

LUNGES: Stand with your feet hip-width apart, with the hand weights in your hands. Step forward with one leg, bending your knee to a ninety-degree angle. Keep your torso erect. Step back to the starting position, then repeat with the other leg.

I don't necessarily do all of these exercises each time I use weights. I mold my routine to meet my needs for that particular week. For example, in a week that I've taken two yoga classes that included a lot of standing poses (which tend to work your butt), I'll skip lunges in my gym workout. If I've done two boxing classes that week, I'll skip some of the chest, shoulder, and bicep work. I do this to avoid overtraining.

And remember, I use weights light enough that I can do at least twelve reps. I'll do up to twenty reps if necessary for the muscle to feel fairly exhausted when I stop. If the muscle doesn't feel exhausted by twenty reps, I'll add a bit more weight for the next set.

3. THREE TO FIVE MINUTES OF ABS— HOLLY'S FAVORITE AB EXERCISES FOR CARVING A SIX-PACK

I don't do tons of abdominal exercises. Instead, I do only a few minutes of the most effective ab exercises, making sure I use proper form. Using proper form is harder. It's much easier to sloppily perform ten minutes of ab exercises than to perform five minutes using correct form. You won't get the tone and definition from the sloppy versions anyway.

I think the three most effective ab exercises for carving a six-pack are the plank, the side plank, and bicycle crunches. Why? Plank is unbeatable for strengthening and toning your entire core, and it works your six-pack muscles (the *rectus abdominus*) like no other exercise. Side plank is spectacular for developing your obliques, those cool muscles that give definition to the sides of your abdomen. And I love bicycle crunches because they bring it all together by working the six-pack muscles and the obliques. These three form the perfect trinity of ab exercises and are the ones I usually do when I am doing my own gym workout.

So for my ab routine, I first hold **PLANK** for one minute. Next I do **SIDE PLANK**, doing one minute on each side. Finally I do **BICYCLE CRUNCHES**, doing fifty repetitions (twenty-five each side). If I am feeling energetic, I will repeat each exercise.

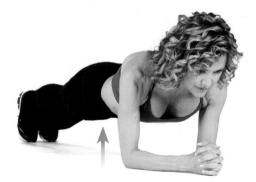

PLANK: Lie flat on your stomach. Prop your upper body up on your forearms. Press into your forearms and lift your knees so your weight is resting on your forearms and toes. Keep your body in a straight line, like a plank of wood. Hold for one minute. (If you can't hold this position for the full minute, drop your knees to the floor for a brief break, then lift again. No sagging in the middle!)

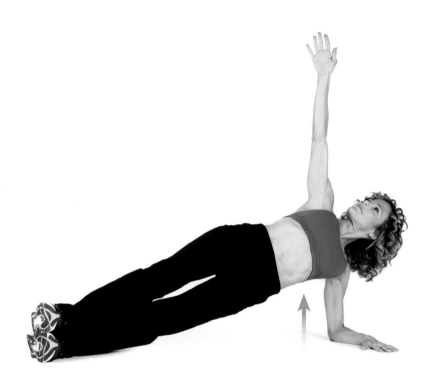

SIDE PLANK: Come into plank. Roll your weight onto your right forearm and the side of your right foot, stacking your left foot on top of your right foot and opening your torso to the left. Lift the left hand toward the ceiling. Keep your body in a straight line. Hold for one minute. (If you can't hold this position for the full minute, lower down for a brief break, then come back up. And just like with plank, no sagging in the middle!) Repeat on the other side.

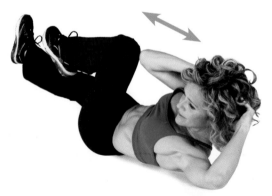

BICYCLE CRUNCHES: Lie on your back. Bring your hands behind your head and lightly place your fingers on each side of your head. Lift your knees so they are straight above your hips. Rotate your torso and bring your right elbow to meet your left knee as you extend your right leg straight out. Now extend your left leg straight out as you rotate your torso to bring your left elbow to meet your right knee. Keep it up, rotating from side to side. Repeat twenty-five times on each side.

HOLLY'S **EXERCISE CLASS** RECOMMENDATIONS

I usually take two or three group exercise classes a week. I love group exercise classes. It is a luxury to have an instructor pushing you, and I enjoy the camaraderie of working out with others. Taking a class with twenty or thirty people motivates me to work a little harder. We feed off each other's energy, making the classes even more fun and challenging.

My favorite classes are cardio boxing and cardio kickboxing. I take them two to three days per week at the gym we own, L.A. Boxing in Lake Forest, California. These classes perfectly implement my workout guidelines, as they include interval cardio along with whole-body resistance training in one viciously efficient workout session.

At L.A. Boxing, the classes are taught by professional and amateur fighters, and they mimic real boxing and kickboxing matches by incorporating three-minute rounds in which you punch or kick a 150-pound hanging Muay Thai bag. These are the most effective classes I've found to get in shape and get shredded fast, and I highly recommend them.

Cardio boxing and kickboxing classes are becoming very popular because of their effective blend of cardio and resistance training, so you can usually find them at your local gym. If possible, join a class in which you are actually punching or kicking a heavy bag (as opposed to hitting and kicking in the air, pretending to hit an opponent or bag). Making actual contact with a heavy bag is excellent resistance training and maximizes your results.

Once in a while I'll do a cardio weight-training class at my local gym. I like classes that combine some cardio with light weight lifting. I also like circuit training classes, especially those that utilize Bosu balls (which are great for working on balance and strengthening the core).

On occasion I will do a spin class, but I get bored with an hour of spinning, and I don't need an hour of high-intensity cardio. If I take a spin class, I sit by the door and leave after about thirty minutes and then finish up with some light weight training or one of my Ten-Minute Yoga Sequences.

HOLLY'S **HOME BOXING** WORKOUT

If you are unable to join a boxing gym, you can do a home boxing workout. I used to do this once or twice a week before we owned our gym. The entire workout takes about thirty-five minutes. All you need is two one-pound hand weights and a jump rope. If you have a timer handy, bring it on. Otherwise, you can just check the clock. You're going to alternate three-minute rounds of jumping rope with three-minute rounds of shadow-boxing drills until you hit a total of thirty minutes. You'll end with three to five minutes of abdominal exercises. This is a well-rounded, all-over body workout that can be performed anywhere, anytime. Blast your music and have fun!

ROUND 1 THREE MINUTES OF JUMPING ROPE TO WARM UP AND START YOUR FOOTWORK

Begin to slowly jump rope, then increase your speed and intensity as your body begins to warm up.

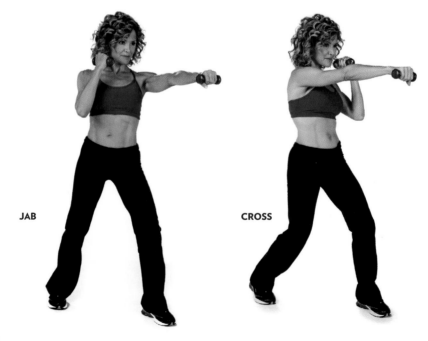

JAB   CROSS

ROUND 2 THREE MINUTES OF SHADOWBOXING

Hold your one-pound hand weights and come into a boxing stance by bending your elbows with the weights near your face, firming your core with your knees slightly bent. Start with a jab (short punch with your left hand), then immediately follow with a cross (punch with your right hand). Get your rhythm down by twisting at your waist as you throw the jab and cross evenly, one after the other with no stopping in between. Make sure to keep your core tight. After you're comfortable with the rhythm, speed it up, but keep the movements even and controlled.

ROUND 3 THREE MINUTES OF JUMPING ROPE

ROUND 4 THREE MINUTES OF ROLLS WITH SHADOWBOXING

Hold your one-pound hand weights and come into a boxing stance. Keeping the feet about hip distance apart, you're going to "roll" from side to side, as if you are ducking a punch. Keep your back straight and perform the roll by bending at your knees (not at the waist). As you roll to the left, rotate your torso so your right shoulder points

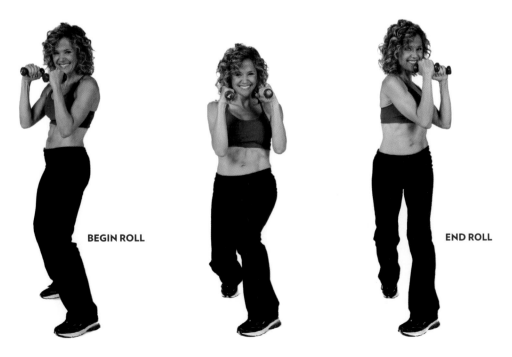

BEGIN ROLL **END ROLL**

in front of you. As you roll to the right, rotate so your left shoulder points in front of you. Keep rolling from side to side without stopping, and increase your speed as you get your rhythm down. Once you have your rhythm, you can up the intensity by adding punches. As you roll to the right, throw a left jab (this will make sense to you as you do it because your left shoulder will be moving forward as you roll to the right). As you roll to the left, throw a right cross. Keep your core firm and keep it going! You ought to be sweating if you're doing it right.

ROUND 5 THREE MINUTES OF JUMPING ROPE

ROUND 6 THREE MINUTES OF SHADOWBOXING

ROUND 7 THREE MINUTES OF JUMPING ROPE

ROUND 8 THREE MINUTES OF ROLLS WITH SHADOWBOXING

ROUND 9 THREE MINUTES OF JUMPING ROPE

ROUND 10 THREE MINUTES OF SHADOWBOXING

End this session with three to five minutes of abdominal exercises. You know my favorites. Do one minute of plank, one minute of side plank (on each side), then end with bicycle crunches (at least fifty).

KICK-START
YOUR EXERCISE PROGRAM!

As I mentioned earlier, Chapter Eleven is going to give you exactly what I did for exercise (and eating) for an entire month. (It also sets forth what I do each morning to set my day up to be peaceful and successful.) Photocopy the chapter. Keep it with you. It will help take all the guesswork out of the plan and let you follow me to success!

PART FOUR

FOLLOW
HOLLY

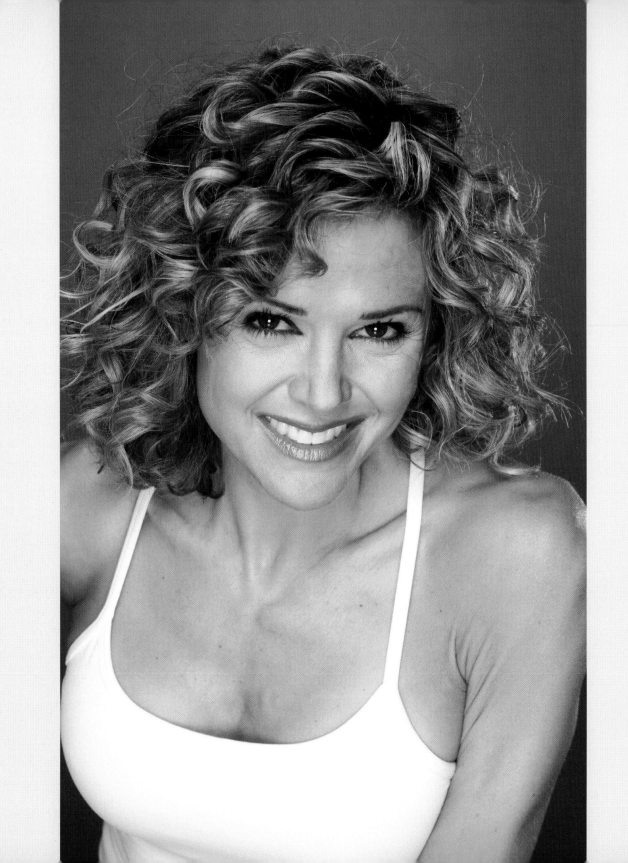

CHAPTER 11

ONE
MONTH
WITH HOLLY

How does all of this work in real life? I'll show you. In this chapter I give you exactly what I did for stress management, eating (pig-outs and all), and exercise each day for one month so you can see how I bring all three components together. Nothing is left out.

I start mentally setting up my day to be peaceful and successful the moment I open my eyes. In the first section, entitled "Holly's Magical Morning Routine," I'll tell you exactly what I do. Then I give you an entire month of what I ate so you see how I apply the eating principles, and you'll become familiar with all of my easy, five-ingredients-or-less, family-friendly recipes. I also list what I did for exercise each day.

You can either follow this exactly (why reinvent the wheel?) or use it as a model to create your own. Here we go!

STRESS MANAGEMENT—HOLLY'S MAGICAL MORNING ROUTINE

People ask me exactly what I do to stay centered in peace each day. I learned, after much trial and error, that what I do first thing in the morning dictates how the rest of my day will go. So I experimented with starting the day with the stress-reduction techniques that are most meaningful to me, and it was like magic. Whenever I established myself in this peaceful state of mind first thing in the morning, my day took on the same uplifted energy that I brought from my morning routine. So now, my morning routine that I developed is sacrosanct. Here's exactly what I do.

FOUR-COUNT BREATH BEGINS MY DAY

As soon as I awaken, before I get out of bed, I start with a few Four-Count Breaths. Then, still lying in bed, I mentally go through a "My Life" statement. This is a statement that I wrote (and continue to annotate), laying out exactly how I want and expect my life to be. It lists my goals, including both the achievements I expect to accomplish and the joy I will experience when and as these things come to pass. It addresses the way I want my body to look and feel, my relationships, my businesses, my finances, my home—everything. It is an uplifting, magical story of my ideal life. It places me in the positive state of mind I intend to have for the day, and it centers me in what is important to me, helping immensely in deciding what I will commit to and participate in each day.

WATER, THEN COFFEE

Next, I get up and drink about twelve ounces of warm water. I learned from Ayurveda and Chinese medicine that warm water first thing in the morning is better for us than cold. I know it feels easier on my system. And I don't know if this is true or not, but I read years ago that drinking water first thing in the morning starts to rev up your metabolism. That would be nice! But in any event, it gives me a head start on my daily water requirement (I like to drink around 60 to 64 ounces to keep water retention at bay), and I swear it has improved my skin.

Next, I go downstairs to the kitchen and make a small cup of espresso. Yum! It's no secret that I love my coffee, but even smelling the grounds as I load the espresso machine makes me smile.

TIME FOR MEDITATION

Cup of coffee in hand, I trot back upstairs for my reading and meditation session. I always sit in the same spot—on my side of the bed, with pillows stacked up behind me to hold my spine erect. I think sitting in the same spot for meditation (whenever possible) is important because after meditating in that same spot for a while, it will trigger your mind to start slowing the thoughts. And the spot gets infused with the best vibes you can experience. Just wait. Others will start commenting that your special place feels very Zen.

I start by reading some inspirational literature for a few minutes (or much longer if I have the time) of any name or nature. I've been doing this for decades, so by now I have a healthy library of all manner of spiritual books. I read them all. The Bible, Ralph Waldo Emerson, Eckhart Tolle, the yoga sutras, Norman Vincent Peale, Wayne Dyer, Ernest Holmes, Venice Bloodworth, Marianne Williamson, Wallace Wattles, the Bhagavad Gita, Joel Goldsmith, Abraham-Hicks books, Louise Hay, Deepak Chopra, and on and on. This reading always uplifts my thought, and while I am reading, I am slowing my breath. By now I am naturally inhaling to at least the count of four and exhaling to at least the count of four (and usually much longer). The thoughts are slowing, and the stillness is starting to envelop me.

Then I meditate. I might take a sentence, or even just one word, from what I've read that morning to focus on, or I might just drop into listening to my slow and resonant breath. My mind quiets. After a brief time, I feel that inner peacefulness. If I have the time to just sit in the peacefulness, it begins to ripen into joy. If I spend time there, the joy opens me to bliss.

On the days I reach that blissful state, I feel like I have touched heaven. I come out of the meditation feeling elevated, enlivened, and inspired to move forward in a noble and uplifted state of mind. It is at this point that I get out my list of goals that I keep in my nightstand, and I slowly read through them, pondering each one, and capturing that internal feeling of what it will feel like when I have achieved that goal. Because I have centered myself in my higher consciousness before this step, this is not an intense, "I'm going to kick butt!" type of feeling or attitude. Instead, it is joy and grateful anticipation, a feeling of kindness and empathy toward myself and others—a soft and lovely feeling.

GET THE CARDIO DONE FIRST THING IF POSSIBLE

After a bit of time spent there (and it can vary from a few moments to minutes to a half hour or more when I have the time), I slowly come out and start to get ready for my day. Many times, if my schedule allows, I'll do my cardio session now. I always find that just getting my cardio done first thing in the morning makes me feel terrific and usually sets me up to be motivated to do some other exercise later in the day, too, like a few minutes of light weights or one of my Ten-Minute Yoga Sequences.

Once I finish that, it's time for a shower, then on to my day.

KEEP THE FOUR-COUNT BREATH GOING

During the day, I have trained myself to do the Four-Count Breath at little intervals throughout the day. When I am driving, I always do the Four-Count Breath at red lights and stop signs. If the phone rings, I do at least one before I pick up the phone. And, of course, whenever I feel a little stress, I use the Four-Count Breath. Gently and easily, I breathe in and out a few times and relax my neck and shoulders, and that takes the edge off.

As I go about my day, I stay alert to maintaining the peaceful center I established first thing that morning. If anything happens that stresses me, I simply use any of the other tools I've given you. One of my favorites is Switch Your Focus. It's quick and very effective for me. No matter what happens during the day, I work to keep my mind on positive things. That is one of my responsibilities to myself—and others.

I found that the more consistent I got with using my favorite stress-reduction techniques, the more quickly effective they became. It makes sense. It's like learning anything else. We want it to become a habit, a new conditioned response whenever anything even starts looking like it's going to go awry. When I first used the Four-Count Breath, sometimes it took me six or more breaths to start feeling some relief. Now it is almost instantaneous. Ahhhh. And it will work for you too.

So now you have my morning routine. This is what I do every day, and it never fails to set me up for a wonderful day and to keep stress at bay.

Now let's get on to eating and exercise, and we'll pull all the elements together.

EATING AND EXERCISE—FOLLOW HOLLY TO KICK-START YOUR WEIGHT LOSS!

Based on my height (five feet two inches) and my activity level (moderate to very active), my daily calorie allotment is 1,700 to 1,800 calories per day to maintain my happy weight of 107 to 108. If I use the eating guidelines and recipes I've developed, this number of calories completely satiates me. And I average about an hour of exercise most days. Some days I exercise more than an hour, and other days much less. I do very occasionally take a day off completely, but generally, at the very least I'll get some walking in. In this section, I list exactly what I ate and what I did for exercise each day for a month.

All the recipes listed on the following pages are included in Chapter Twelve. I recommend that you follow me for one month to acclimate to the plan, get trained on the correct balance of protein, carbs, and fat, and learn the easy recipes. In the recipes, I include where to buy certain foods (generally, Costco, Trader Joe's, or a regular grocery store).

This will also help to entrench you in your new eating habits without your having to think too hard. Once you see how easy this is, you won't have any problem using the guidelines I have given you to personalize the program to meet your natural appetite patterns and palate. That's what I do, and that's why I am off the diet roller coaster once and for all—I'm not missing out on anything I love to eat.

A word of caution: You must measure your portions. Even to this day, I still measure out the ingredients in my recipes because, to be frank, my eyeballing of "proper portion" size changes depending on how hungry I am.

As for exercise, remember, variety of activity is the key. So if you like to play tennis, swim, cycle, jog, garden (I always break a sweat), walk on the beach . . . those count toward your exercise for the day. Just keep moving in whatever way makes you happy!

So use the following month of menus and workouts to follow me exactly, or as a tool to inspire you and plan your own meals and workouts for the month. Let's get started!

HOLLY'S MONTH OF MENUS AND WORKOUTS

DAY 1

BREAKFAST:	Holly's Cheese Blintzes/coffee
LUNCH:	Holly's Terrific Tuna Sandwich/apple/hot tea
SNACK:	Almonds (100 calories' worth)
DINNER:	Holly's Rotisserie Chicken with Salsa/half of a baked potato/Holly's Salad/hot tea
EXERCISE:	Twenty-two minutes of interval cardio on the elliptical machine, then five minutes on the stationary bike, followed by five minutes on the rowing machine

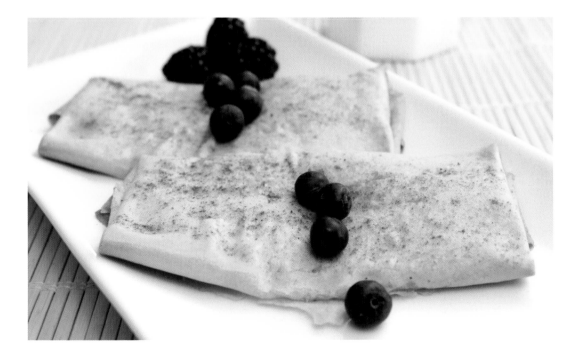

DAY 2

BREAKFAST:	Holly's Cheese Blintzes/coffee
LUNCH:	Holly's Turkey and Cheese Pita/carrot sticks/hot tea
SNACK:	Apple
DINNER:	Holly's Cinnamon Salmon/Holly's Roasted Veggies/Holly's Salad/Crystal Light lemonade
EXERCISE:	One-hour cardio boxing class at L.A. Boxing

DAY 3

BREAKFAST:	Holly's Cottage Cheese Sundae/coffee
LUNCH:	Holly's Folded P.B. Sandwich/apple/hot tea
SNACK:	Strawberries

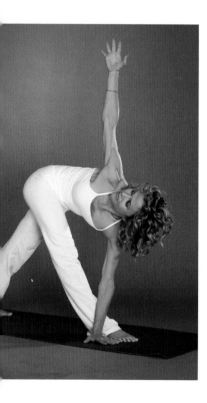

DINNER: Holly's Curry Chicken Breasts/Holly's Spicy Green Beans/Holly's Salad/small glass of wine

EXERCISE: Gym workout—twenty minutes of interval cardio on the elliptical machine, then ten minutes on the VersaClimber, followed by fifteen minutes of all-over-body light weight training, then three minutes of abs

DAY 4

BREAKFAST:	Holly's Lemon Bagel/coffee
LUNCH:	Holly's Cottage Cheese Potato/hot tea
SNACK:	Apple
DINNER:	Holly's Cheesy Chicken/Holly's Broiled Tomatoes/Holly's Microwave Cauliflower/Diet 7-Up
EXERCISE:	A.M.: One-hour cardio boxing class at L.A. Boxing; P.M.: My Beginner's Ten-Minute Yoga Sequence

DAY 5

BREAKFAST:	Holly's Cheese Blintzes/coffee
LUNCH:	Holly's Tortilla Wrap/Leftover Holly's Broiled Tomatoes/cucumber spears/hot tea
SNACK:	Pear
DINNER:	Holly's Shrimp with Thai Noodles/Holly's Salad/hot tea
EXERCISE:	Twenty-two minutes of interval cardio on the elliptical machine, then five minutes on the VersaClimber, followed by five minutes on the rowing machine (I'm really liking the rowing machine. It's efficient. If you firm your core a bit when you row, you'll work your abs as well as your glutes and legs.)

DAY 6

BREAKFAST:	Holly's Scrambled Egg Blintz/coffee
LUNCH:	Holly's Tofu Sandwich/carrot sticks/hot tea
SNACK:	Apple
DINNER:	Holly's Spaghetti and Meatballs/Holly's Salad/ small glass of wine
EXERCISE:	Spin class (thirty minutes), then my Advanced Ten-Minute Yoga Sequence

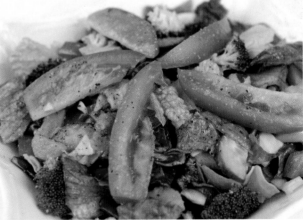

DAY 7

BREAKFAST: Holly's Breakfast Parfait/coffee

LUNCH: Holly's Turkey and Cheese Pita/
bell pepper strips/hot tea

SNACK: Pear

DINNER: Pig out! We went to a restaurant, and I
had a hamburger, fries, a Diet Coke, and
a small chocolate shake. Yum!

EXERCISE: I hiked Squaw Peak in Phoenix, Arizona. It
was awesome! It took a total of one hour.

DAY 8

BREAKFAST: Zone bar/coffee

LUNCH: Holly's Cottage Cheese and Fruit Salad/hot tea

SNACK: None—I ate a little lighter and had fewer carbs
today, which I frequently do the day after a
high-carb pig-out like I had yesterday.

DINNER: I had my typical day-after-pig-out dinner—I
stir-fried a big batch of frozen green veggies
and baked a large piece of salmon/hot tea

EXERCISE: A.M.: Gym workout—thirty-three minutes of interval
cardio on the elliptical machine, followed by fifteen
minutes of all over-body light weight training, then
three minutes of abs
P.M.: Walked two miles (I did this extra cardio
today because of yesterday's pig-out. I usually do
some easy extra cardio the day after a pig-out.)

DAY 9

BREAKFAST:	Holly's Sunrise Sandwich/coffee
LUNCH:	Holly's Terrific Tuna Sandwich/apple/hot tea
SNACK:	Pear
DINNER:	Holly's Rotisserie Chicken with Salsa/Holly's Roasted Veggies/Holly's Salad/Crystal Light lemonade
EXERCISE:	I took a one-hour water aerobics class with my daughter. We laughed hysterically, but it was tough! What a great way to add variety to my workouts.

DAY 10

BREAKFAST:	Holly's Cottage Cheese Berry Delight/coffee
LUNCH:	Holly's Pita Pizza Taco (using leftover Holly's Roasted Veggies from dinner the previous night)/cucumber spears/hot tea
SNACK:	Apple
DINNER:	Holly's Nachos/Holly's Salad/Crystal Light iced tea
EXERCISE:	Ninety-minute wilderness hike

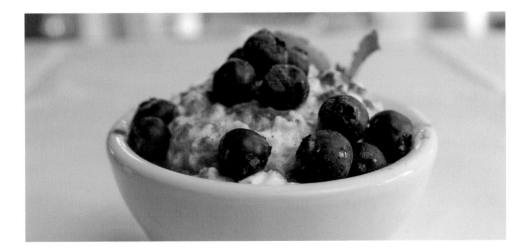

DAY 11

BREAKFAST:	Holly's Cheese Blintzes/coffee
LUNCH:	Holly's Tofu Sandwich/carrot sticks/hot tea
SNACK:	Apple
DINNER:	One pint of nonfat frozen yogurt (approximately 500 calories) with one serving of peanut M&M's (250 calories)/decaf coffee
EXERCISE:	A.M.: Walk two miles
	P.M.: Walk two miles

DAY 12

BREAKFAST:	Holly's Cottage Cheese Sundae/coffee
LUNCH:	Holly's Egg Salad Sandwich/carrot sticks/hot tea
SNACK:	Apple
DINNER:	Holly's Stuffed Baked Potato/Holly's Salad/hot tea
EXERCISE:	A.M.: Iyengar yoga class
	P.M.: Twenty-five minutes of interval cardio on the elliptical machine

DAY 13

BREAKFAST:	Holly's Breakfast Parfait/coffee
LUNCH:	I was at the Cheesecake Factory. I ordered the salmon salad with dressing on the side and hot tea. This was a perfect choice—a large piece of poached salmon on a bed of greens.

SNACK:	Two pieces of Hershey's sugar-free dark chocolate They are thirty calories each (and really good).
DINNER:	Holly's High-Protein Burger and Veggies/ Holly's Salad/Crystal Light lemonade
EXERCISE:	One-hour cardio kickboxing class at L.A. Boxing

DAY 14

BREAKFAST:	Holly's Cheese Blintzes/coffee
LUNCH:	Holly's Turkey and Cheese Pita/carrot sticks/hot tea
SNACK:	Apple
DINNER:	Pig out! We went out for pizza, then stopped to get ice cream (I had a double cone—yum!).
EXERCISE:	Gym workout—twenty-two minutes of interval cardio on the elliptical machine followed by eight minutes on the rowing machine; fifteen minutes of all-over-body light weight training, four minutes of abs, and five minutes of stretching

DAY 15

BREAKFAST:	Zone bar/coffee
LUNCH:	Holly's Cottage Cheese Berry Delight/decaf coffee
SNACK:	None (I generally eat a bit lighter the day after a pig-out. I find I usually don't have much of an appetite.)
DINNER:	Holly's Grilled Salmon/small yam sprinkled with cinnamon and Splenda/ Holly's Roasted Veggies/hot tea
EXERCISE:	A.M.: Walked two miles P.M.: Spin class (I left after thirty-five minutes)

DAY 16

BREAKFAST: Holly's Veggie Omelet/coffee

LUNCH: Half of a Baja Fresh Chicken Burrito Ultimo (no guacamole or sour cream)/a mound of fresh salsa/iced tea (I took the other half of the burrito home to have for lunch the next day)

SNACK: Pear

DINNER: Holly's Curry Chicken Breasts/Holly's French Fries/Holly's Salad/hot tea

EXERCISE: A.M.: I took a one-hour circuit-training group exercise class at the local gym.

P.M.: Ninety-minute restorative yoga class (Restorative yoga does not count as exercise. It is the mildest of the mild yoga classes. It is fantastic to reduce stress and replenish you mentally and physically. I have found the stress-reduction effect definitely helps cut cravings.)

DAY 17

BREAKFAST: Holly's Cottage Cheese Sundae/coffee

LUNCH: The other half of the Baja Fresh Chicken Burrito Ultimo from lunch the day before (no guacamole or sour cream)/a mound of fresh salsa/hot tea

SNACK: Apple

DINNER: Holly's Grilled Steak/Holly's Broiled Tomatoes/Holly's Stir-Fried Asparagus/Holly's Salad/small glass of wine

EXERCISE: I took the day off.

DAY 18

BREAKFAST: Holly's Lemon Bagel/coffee

LUNCH: Holly's Tofu Sandwich/carrot sticks/hot tea

SNACK: Apple

DINNER: Half of a Trader Joe's truffle pizza/Holly's Salad/ hot tea (Trader Joe's has a great selection of frozen pizzas, and most are on flatbread so the calories and carb content are lower. I haven't had a bad one yet.) This half of a pizza was 390 calories, and I added one ounce of low-fat mozzarella for an additional eighty calories, and boy, was it good!

EXERCISE: A.M.: Iyengar yoga class (This was a very mild class. We did all of the poses sitting on the floor.)

P.M.: One-hour cardio boxing class at L.A. Boxing

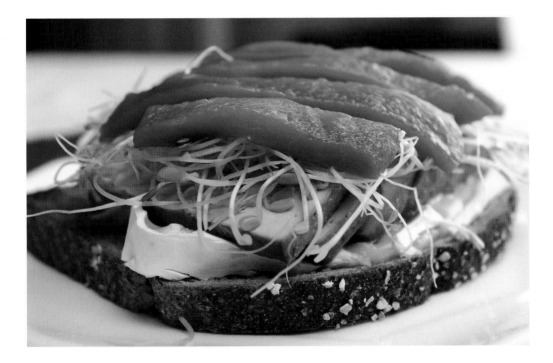

DAY 19

BREAKFAST: Holly's Lemon Bagel/coffee

LUNCH: I went to Subway for lunch. I had a turkey and cheese sandwich from the low-calorie menu (about 500 calories)/iced tea

SNACK: Strawberries

DINNER: Half of a frozen Trader Joe's truffle pizza (I had the first half the night before)/Holly's Microwave Cauliflower/Holly's Stir-Fried Cabbage/hot tea

EXERCISE: I had jury duty today, so I just walked on our breaks. I took my pedometer with me in my purse so I could measure my walks. I ended up walking about three miles total! Not bad. (I frequently take a pedometer with me on days like this when I won't have time for a formal exercise session. Just having the pedometer with me reminds me to walk when I can, and I am always pleasantly surprised at how it adds up.)

DAY 20

BREAKFAST: Holly's Egg and Bacon Sandwich/coffee

LUNCH: Holly's Cottage Cheese and Fruit Salad/hot tea

SNACK: Almonds (100 calories' worth)

DINNER: One pint of nonfat frozen yogurt (approximately 500 calories) with one serving of peanut M&M's (250 calories)/decaf coffee

EXERCISE: Gym workout—thirty-five minutes of interval cardio on the stationary bike followed by fifteen minutes of all-over-body light weight training, then four minutes of abs

DAY 21

BREAKFAST:	Holly's Cheese Blintzes/coffee
LUNCH:	Pig out! What can I say? I skipped "lunch" and instead had a big old bowl of Dreyer's peanut butter and chocolate chunk ice cream, and I added some extra dark chocolate chips and whipped cream. Ridiculously good!
SNACK:	None
DINNER:	Just a small portion of cheese and crackers and an apple (about 500 calories total); not a great eating day, but I'll get back on track tomorrow
EXERCISE:	One-hour cardio kickboxing class at L.A. Boxing

DAY 22

BREAKFAST:	Holly's Breakfast Parfait/coffee
LUNCH:	Holly's Pita Pizza Taco/carrot sticks/hot tea
SNACK:	None
DINNER:	Holly's Fajita Salad/hot tea
EXERCISE:	A.M.: Forty-five minutes of interval cardio on the recumbent stationary bike
	P.M.: My Advanced Ten-Minute Yoga Sequence

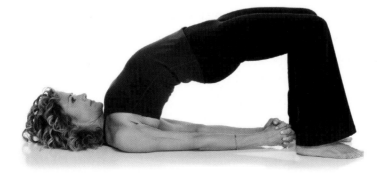

DAY 23

BREAKFAST:	Premier Protein bar (270 calories and thirty grams of protein)/coffee
LUNCH:	Holly's Tortilla Wrap/small salad/hot tea
SNACK:	Bell pepper strips/light ranch dressing
DINNER:	We went to Flame Broiler fast-food restaurant. Flame Broiler is *awesome*. It's topped all kinds of lists for being an excellent "healthy" restaurant, and the food is really good. I got the Chicken Veggie Bowl with brown rice (650 calories according to their nutrition information, and that seemed about right)/iced tea
EXERCISE:	One-hour athletic conditioning class at the local gym. We used hand weights, a barbell, a Bosu fitness ball, and the step to go through a fast-paced, high-rep resistance workout that targeted every area of the body.

DAY 24

BREAKFAST:	Holly's Cottage Cheese Berry Delight/coffee
LUNCH:	Holly's Folded P.B. Sandwich/apple/hot tea
SNACK:	Pear
DINNER:	Holly's Thousand Island Chicken/ Holly's Rice/Holly's Salad/hot tea
EXERCISE:	A.M.: Thirty-three minutes of interval cardio on the recumbent stationary bike P.M.: Ninety-minute restorative yoga class (Remember—this doesn't count as exercise. It is, however, one of the most effective stress reducers I have found.)

DAY 25

BREAKFAST:	Holly's Sunrise Sandwich/coffee
LUNCH:	Holly's Terrific Tuna Sandwich/apple/hot tea
SNACK:	Strawberries
DINNER:	Holly's Grilled Steak/Holly's Sautéed Spinach/ Holly's Salad/Crystal Light lemonade
EXERCISE:	A.M.: My Intermediate Ten-Minute Yoga Sequence P.M.: One-hour cardio boxing class at L.A. Boxing

DAY 26

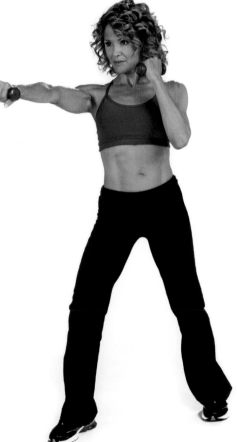

BREAKFAST:	Holly's Cottage Cheese Berry Delight/coffee
LUNCH:	Holly's Folded P.B. Sandwich/ apple/hot tea
SNACK:	Pear
DINNER:	Holly's Baked Pork Chops/ Holly's Baked Apples/Holly's Rice/Crystal Light lemonade
EXERCISE:	A.M.: Twenty-five minutes of interval cardio on the upright stationary bike followed by eight minutes on the VersaClimber P.M.: My Beginner Ten-Minute Yoga Sequence

DAY 27

BREAKFAST: I had one of the leftover Holly's Baked Apples and added one cup of low-fat cottage cheese—tasty!/coffee

LUNCH: Holly's Tofu Sandwich/small salad/hot tea

SNACK: Apple

DINNER: Stuffed salmon from Costco (this is a six-ounce fresh salmon fillet filled with about three ounces of crab and rice)/Holly's Roasted Veggies/Holly's Salad/glass of Cabernet

EXERCISE: A.M.: Twenty-five minutes of interval cardio on the recumbent stationary bike

P.M.: Ninety-minute Vinyasa flow yoga class (this was a fairly mild class)

DAY 28

BREAKFAST: Holly's Cheese Blintzes/coffee

LUNCH: Lean Cuisine Four Cheese Cannelloni/veggies and low-fat ranch dip/hot tea

SNACK: Apple

DINNER: Holly's Cheesy Chicken/Holly's Stir-Fried Zucchini/Holly's Salad/hot tea

EXERCISE: A.M.: Walked four miles

P.M.: My Advanced Ten-Minute Yoga Sequence

DAY 29

BREAKFAST:	Holly's Cottage Cheese Sundae/coffee
LUNCH:	Holly's Terrific Tuna Sandwich/apple/Diet 7-Up
SNACK:	None
DINNER:	Pig out! We had pizza night, but I didn't completely go overboard. I took two slices of cheese pizza, took the topping off of one of the slices and added it to the other, then threw away the crust from the second piece. That made one nice-sized piece of "double-loaded" cheese pizza which totally satisfied me (and didn't have so many carbs), along with Holly's Roasted Veggies/Holly's Salad/small glass of wine/small bowl of cookie-dough ice cream for dessert
EXERCISE:	One-hour cardio boxing class at L.A. Boxing

DAY 30

BREAKFAST:	Zone bar/coffee
LUNCH:	Holly's Turkey and Cheese Pita/carrot sticks/hot tea
SNACK:	None
DINNER:	Holly's Thousand Island Chicken/Holly's Spicy Green Beans/Holly's Salad/hot tea
EXERCISE:	A.M.: Twenty-five-minute jog/run (I alternated three minutes of jogging with thirty to forty-five seconds of running) P.M.: Iyengar yoga class

DAY 31

BREAKFAST:	Half of a bagel-shop egg sandwich (half a honey wheat bagel, one egg, one ounce cheddar cheese)/coffee
LUNCH:	I was at an event at which they served food. I had a roast beef sandwich—I removed the top slice of bread and folded it in half (no mayo, just mustard)/salad/decaf coffee
SNACK:	Melon slices (served at the event)/hot tea
DINNER:	Holly's Nachos/Holly's Salad/Crystal Light lemonade
EXERCISE:	I took a day off from formal exercise. I just walked the dog for thirty minutes in the early evening.

THE FORMULA FOR A HEALTHY MIND, HEALTHY BODY, AND HEALTHY LIFE

Plan a morning routine that works to center you in peace and happy anticipation for what the day will offer. You want to have such a ritual first thing in the morning so you proactively place yourself in a positive, uplifted state of mind *before* you start your day. It is your state of mind that will determine how you react to every event of the day and how much or how little stress you have. So I think having a morning routine is critical. It is so much harder to pull yourself up later in the day after you are tired and have maybe faced some stuff that didn't please you. Establish your foundation of peace before you step out the door. Besides, it makes life so much fun!

I know this is not always easy. I hear you. I remember years ago when I would dread the moment my eyes would open in the morning because I just couldn't face another day of what felt like hell: the strain of dealing with uncooperative kids, ex-spouses, my job, trying to blend a family, terrible fatigue that I couldn't shake—being tugged by all kinds of demands that I couldn't begin to satisfy, much less find enjoyment for myself. I began and ended my days in despair. The cycle just continued until I made a decision to take control of my thoughts. Those new thoughts created new, positive emotions. And now, well, I can't imagine living as I used to. It was so unnecessary! There was nothing to stop me but myself.

You'll find the eating plan simple and delicious. It delivers on my promise that the recipes are family-friendly. Pick a dozen or so of your favorites, make those your staples, and sprinkle in some of the others for variety. This will lighten your grocery-shopping load as well, saving you time and money. I've listed more than 50 of my favorite recipes in the next chapter.

As for exercise, just get out there and move every day in a way that makes you happy! Remember when we were kids and we moved all day long? We didn't have just one defined hour of exercise and then tell the other kids, "Nope! That's it! I've played for my hour today. I'm sitting down the rest of the day." Heck, no! We ran around on and off all day, following the fun. Yet as adults we sit glued to our computers and televisions or driving our cars for hours on end—and then we wonder why we're gaining weight.

Wait till you see how good you're going to feel when you bring these three elements together. As you apply the stress-management tools and find yourself in control of your emotions and moods, your stress will decrease. Without that uncontrolled stress spiking your appetite, control over your eating will be handed over to you. And without all that stress and anxiety robbing you of your energy, exercising every day won't feel like a chore. You'll want to move! And then, my friends, you'll receive the best gift anyone could give you: You'll recapture that youthful vitality and excitement about your future. We're not old until we stop moving forward.

Today I am exuberant about life. I am so grateful for everything I have and eagerly anticipate more. It is the best possible way to go through life. Come on. Join me. Let's do this together. Why should I have all the fun?

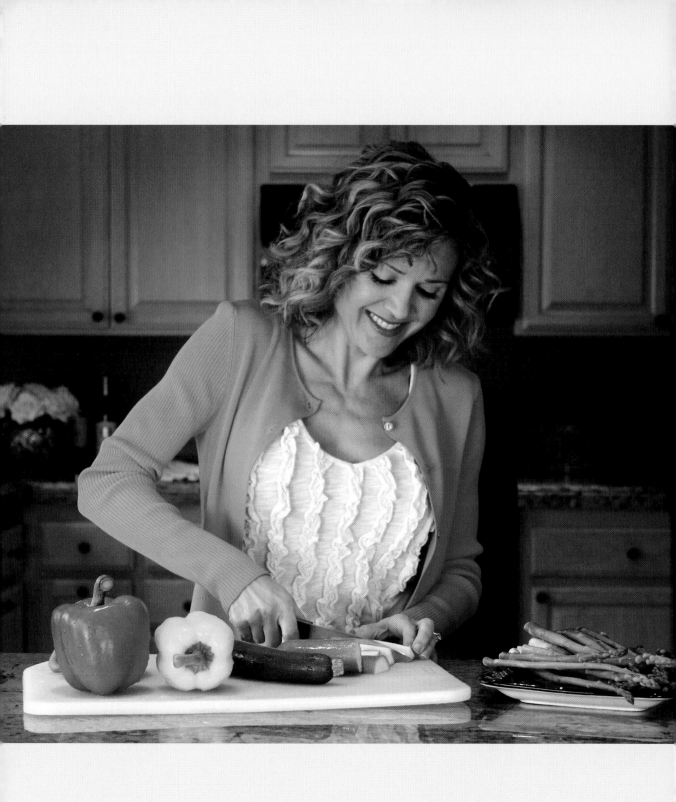

CHAPTER 12

HOLLY'S RECIPES

I don't have the time or patience to do a lot of exotic cooking. Although I appreciate a good meal, I know I will never consistently stick to any eating program that requires me to follow detailed recipes and use ingredients my family and I aren't used to.

Simple is my mantra. Almost all of my recipes use five ingredients or fewer (excluding salt and pepper), and many times combine pre-made or precooked items with new ingredients to create quick, easy, healthy meals that everyone in our family will eat and enjoy.

I eat regular, everyday foods that you'll find in your local grocery store: tuna, peanut butter, pizza, nachos, chicken, and salads. I won't eat "diet" foods or nonfat foods that, to me, are just weird and tasteless. Veggie recipes don't get any easier than mine, and the kids love them.

You'll enjoy the recipe photos. I prepared the food myself, exactly as I always do (no tricks or additions or food stylists to make the foods look more perfect), and my husband took the photos in our kitchen (then he ate the props). I did this so you can see what the recipes really look like when you make them at home yourself. I think they make a beautiful presentation, good enough to impress any guest. Best of all? These recipes are all quick. Have fun with them. Change them up to meet your tastes.

HOLLY'S BREAKFAST RECIPES

Each recipe is an individual serving, unless otherwise noted. The descriptions often specify the brands I use, but you can substitute other brands. Be sure to check the calorie count on a substituted brand, as it may vary from the one listed.

HOLLY'S BREAKFAST PARFAIT

|| APPROXIMATELY 290 CALORIES ||

* 1 container Yoplait Light nonfat yogurt
* 1 cup high-fiber, high-protein cereal

Pour 1 container of Yoplait Light nonfat yogurt into a bowl. Stir in 1 serving of a high-fiber, high-protein cereal. (I like Nature's Path Organic Optimum Power cereal. A 1-cup serving contains 190 calories and 9 grams of protein.)

HOLLY'S COTTAGE CHEESE SUNDAE

|| APPROXIMATELY 370 CALORIES ||

* 1 cup low-fat cottage cheese
* 1/4 cup raisins
* 1 tbsp honey
* cinnamon

Measure 1 cup of low-fat cottage cheese into a bowl. Add ¼ cup of raisins (130 calories). Drizzle 1 tablespoon of honey over the top and sprinkle with cinnamon. This tastes like something you shouldn't be eating! For fewer calories, reduce the amount of cottage cheese and/or raisins, or substitute 1 or 2 packages of Splenda for the honey.

HOLLY'S FRENCH TOAST OMELET

|| APPROXIMATELY 300 CALORIES ||

* 2 large eggs
* 2 tbsp low-fat milk
* cinnamon
* sweetener (like Splenda)
* powdered sugar
* vanilla (optional)
* 1 piece whole-grain bread
* cooking spray

Beat 2 large eggs with 2 tablespoons of low-fat milk. Add cinnamon and sweetener to taste (I use Splenda). You can add a dash of vanilla, if desired. Soak 1 piece of whole-grain bread in the mixture, turning it over until the bread is completely coated. Pour the bread and egg mixture into a small frying pan sprayed with cooking spray, cover, and cook on medium heat. Flip it over after about 2 or 3 minutes. Cook for another 1 to 2 minutes. Serve with extra cinnamon and a dash of powdered sugar. Delicious!

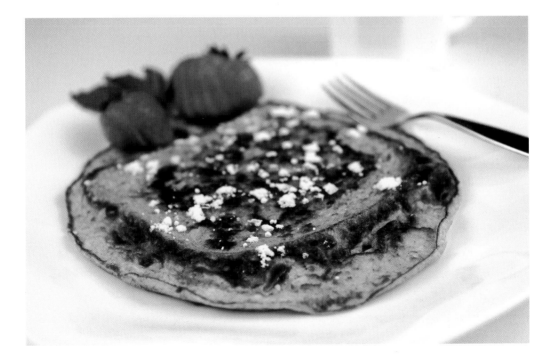

HOLLY'S COTTAGE CHEESE BERRY DELIGHT

‖ APPROXIMATELY 250 CALORIES ‖

* 1 cup low-fat cottage cheese
* sweetener (like Splenda)
* 1/2 cup berries
* cinnamon

Measure 1 cup of low-fat cottage cheese into a bowl. Add approximately ½ cup of berries of your choice, such as strawberries or blueberries. Sprinkle Splenda and cinnamon over the top and serve.

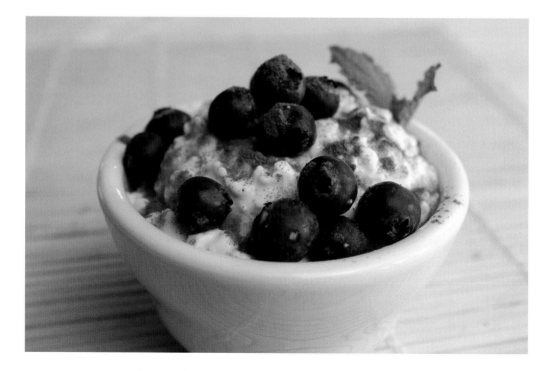

HOLLY'S SUNRISE SANDWICH

|| APPROXIMATELY 270 CALORIES ||

* 2 eggs
* 1/2 Thomas' whole-wheat bagel
* salt
* pepper
* apple cider vinegar (optional)

Poach 2 eggs in a microwave egg poacher. (You can purchase one anywhere that carries housewares, such as Bed Bath & Beyond, Target, Walmart, or even your grocery store.) Toast half of a Thomas' whole-wheat bagel. (These are 240 calories and are presliced. Half is 120 calories.) Put the eggs on the bagel and serve open-faced. Add salt and pepper to taste, or sprinkle it with apple cider vinegar. For those who need more calories at breakfast, my husband loves these topped with a slice of cheddar cheese, which adds approximately 100 calories.

The key to getting the eggs to poach rather than explode in your microwave is to spray the egg holders with cooking spray, then fill them with about ½ inch of water. Break the raw eggs into the cups and break the yolks before microwaving. I also place a microwave food cover over the egg poacher before cooking so if the poacher pops open, I don't have a big mess in my microwave.

HOLLY'S EGG AND BACON SANDWICH

APPROXIMATELY 240 CALORIES

* 1 Thomas' Light Multi-Grain English muffin
* 2 pieces turkey bacon
* 1 egg

Toast 1 Thomas' Light Multi-Grain English muffin. Heat 2 pieces of turkey bacon on a paper towel in the microwave. Poach or scramble 1 egg. Make the sandwich by stacking one piece of turkey bacon on the English muffin, then the egg, then the second piece of bacon, then the top of the muffin. Delicious!

HOLLY'S VEGGIE OMELET

|| APPROXIMATELY 300 CALORIES ||

* 2 eggs
* 2 tbsp low-fat milk
* salt
* pepper

* Holly's Roasted Veggies (see Side Dishes)
* cooking spray
* 1 slice of cheese

Beat 2 eggs with 2 tablespoons of low-fat milk. Add salt and pepper to taste. Stir in leftover Holly's Roasted Veggies (see Side Dishes). Pour into a hot skillet sprayed with cooking spray. Flip when lightly browned on one side. Add 1 slice of cheese to the top. When completely cooked, fold in half and serve. If you have more calories available, you can add a second slice of cheese (approximately 100 calories). I do this for my husband, who gets more calories than I do.

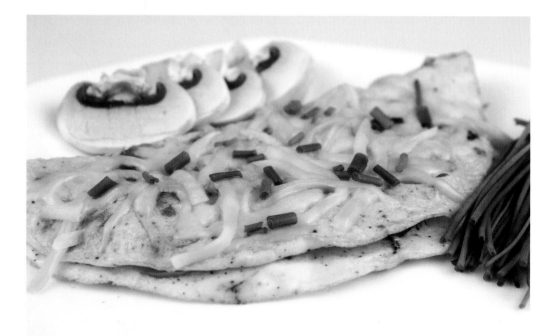

HOLLY'S SCRAMBLED EGG BLINTZ

|| APPROXIMATELY 315 CALORIES ||

* 2 eggs
* salt
* pepper
* 1 oz grated cheese
* 1 crepe

Preheat oven to 350°F. Crack 2 eggs into a bowl and whisk them with salt and pepper. Place the bowl in the microwave, cover, and cook on high for about 1 to 2 minutes, until the eggs are cooked. Stir them with a fork to scramble them. Put 1 ounce of grated cheese in the middle of a crepe. Spoon the scrambled eggs over the cheese, fold the crepe up at both ends, and roll it like a burrito. Bake for 7 to 10 minutes until brown. Tasty!

HOLLY'S LEMON BAGEL

|| APPROXIMATELY 280 CALORIES ||

* 1/2 Thomas' whole-wheat bagel
* 1 tbsp light cream cheese
* 1 egg, hard-boiled
* 1/2 of a small tomato, sliced
* fresh-squeezed lemon juice

Toast half of a Thomas' whole-wheat bagel, then spread it with 1 tablespoon of light cream cheese. Cut 1 hard-boiled egg into slices, and layer them on top of the cream cheese. Top with tomato slices, then squeeze fresh lemon over the top. This is unusual and delicious! If you don't have fresh lemon, you can substitute lemon pepper.

HOLLY'S CHEESE BLINTZES

|| APPROXIMATELY 270 CALORIES ||

* 2/3 cup low-fat ricotta
* 1/2 tsp cinnamon
* vanilla
* 2 pkgs sweetener (Splenda)

* 2 crepes
* cooking spray
* pumpkin pie spice (optional)

Preheat the oven to 350°F. In a bowl, mix ⅔ cup of low-fat ricotta with about ½ teaspoon of cinnamon, a dash of vanilla, and 2 packages of Splenda. (Do not use part-skim ricotta—it is much higher in calories and fat.) Lay 2 crepes out on a cookie sheet lightly sprayed with cooking spray. (I find crepes at the grocery store, usually near the fruit. They are generally about 60 calories each.) Spoon half of the ricotta mixture into the middle of each crepe, fold both ends of the crepe in, and roll each crepe like a burrito. Sprinkle cinnamon sugar or pumpkin pie spice on top of both blintzes. Bake for about 10 minutes, or until lightly browned. These are to die for! And if you enjoy them with hot coffee, this breakfast will keep you full for about 3 or 4 hours!

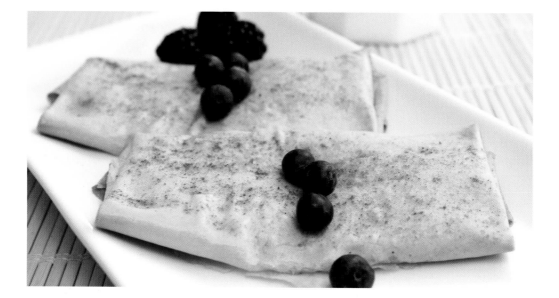

HOLLY'S LOX AND CREAM CHEESE ON A BAGEL

|| APPROXIMATELY 370 CALORIES ||

* 1 onion bagel (trenched)
* 1 tbsp light cream cheese
* 3 oz lox (cured salmon fillet)

Many people enjoy lox and cream cheese on a bagel on weekend mornings, and it just isn't the same on only half a bagel. Instead, cut an onion bagel in half, then "trench out" the bagel by pulling out the soft middle and leaving the harder shell that has the onion and seasoning. This gets rid of about half the bagel, so you're only actually eating half. Spread a thin layer of light cream cheese in the trench, and fill it with about 3 ounces of lox (a little smaller than the palm of your hand). It is easy to do this at a restaurant too. You can do it with any bagel you order that has the flavoring on the outside.

HOLLY'S PITA SCRAMBLE

|| APPROXIMATELY 320 CALORIES ||

* 2 eggs
* 1/2 whole-wheat pita bread
* 1 slice cheddar cheese

Scramble 2 eggs. Heat half of a whole-wheat pita in the microwave for 10 seconds. Put 1 slice of cheddar cheese in the pita, then stuff it with the scrambled eggs. Quick and tasty!

HOLLY'S LUNCH RECIPES

I f you need to cut the calories, you can always serve any of the sandwiches open-faced on 1 slice of bread or stuffed into half a pita (about 80 calories). If you need more calories, just add the second slice of bread, use the whole pita, or add a slice of cheese or extra meat. This is usually necessary for men, whose calorie requirements are generally higher. The calorie counts for each lunch recipe are based on the number of bread slices listed in that recipe.

HOLLY'S FOLDED P.B. SANDWICH

|| **APPROXIMATELY 475 CALORIES (WITH THE APPLE)** ||

* 3 tbsp crunchy peanut butter
* 1 slice whole-grain bread
* 1 medium-sized apple

Spread 3 level tablespoons of crunchy peanut butter on 1 slice of whole-grain bread. Fold in half. Eat with a medium-sized apple. This is very filling, especially if you pair it with hot tea or coffee, and it travels well.

HOLLY'S TOFU SANDWICH

|| APPROXIMATELY 425 CALORIES ||

* 1 piece whole-grain bread
* 1/2 pkg Trader Joe's organic baked tofu
* 1 oz Brie
* spicy peppers
* alfalfa sprouts
* thin-sliced dill pickles (optional)

Toast 1 piece of whole-grain bread. Thinly slice half a package of Trader Joe's organic baked tofu. (My favorite is teriyaki-flavored—it's 150 calories per half package, which is 1 block of tofu.) Thinly slice about 1 ounce of Brie or any cheese you have on hand (light Brie works well too). Place the cheese on the toast while it's hot, so the cheese melts. Add the tofu slices, then top with spicy peppers, alfalfa sprouts, or thinly sliced dill sandwich pickles. My husband doesn't like tofu, but he likes this!

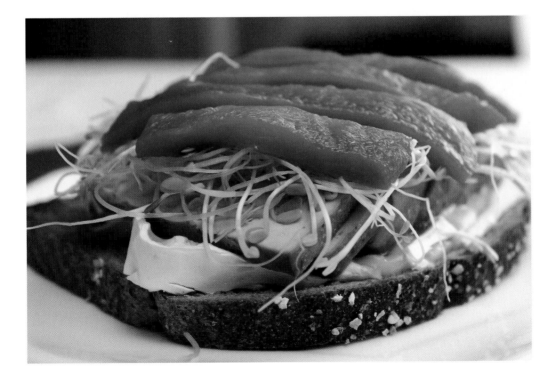

HOLLY'S TERRIFIC TUNA SANDWICH

|| APPROXIMATELY 490 CALORIES ||

* 1 can tuna in water
* 1 medium apple
* 2 slices whole-grain bread

* 1 tbsp reduced-fat canola mayonnaise
* lemon juice, to taste
* garlic salt, to taste

Drain the liquid from a can of tuna packed in water and empty the tuna into a small bowl. Finely chop half of a medium-sized apple and stir into the tuna. Add 1 level tablespoon of canola mayonnaise (the reduced-fat versions taste great and save calories), plus lemon juice and garlic salt to taste. Use 2 slices of whole-grain bread. This tastes best if you toast the bread. To cut the calories, use only 1 slice of bread and eat open-faced, or stuff into half a pita.

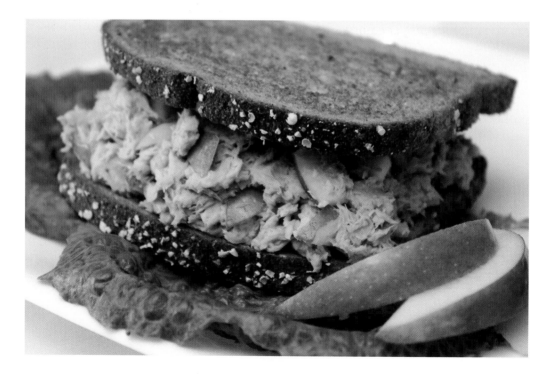

HOLLY'S TURKEY AND CHEESE PITA

|| APPROXIMATELY 430 CALORIES ||

* 1/2 whole-wheat pita bread
* 1 tbsp reduced-fat canola mayonnaise
* 4–5 slices turkey
* 1 slice cheese
* 2–3 lettuce leaves
* 1/2 tomato
* alfalfa sprouts

Cut a whole-wheat pita in half (and use just half unless you need the extra calories). Spread 1 level tablespoon of reduced-fat canola mayonnaise in it, then add 4 or 5 slices of turkey. I like the thin-sliced turkey from the deli counter at the local grocery store. A thin slice of turkey is about 30 calories, so add the amount you can for your proper calorie count. Add a slice of cheese (approximately 100 calories per slice), then lettuce, tomato, and alfalfa sprouts. This is an easy lunch to take to work or school. To cut the calories, omit the mayo (I frequently do, and I don't miss it) and use mustard instead.

HOLLY'S EGG SALAD SANDWICH

|| APPROXIMATELY 420 CALORIES ||

* 2 eggs, hard-boiled
* 1 tbsp reduced-fat canola mayonnaise
* salt and pepper, to taste
* 2 slices whole-grain bread

Mash 2 hard-boiled eggs with 1 tablespoon of reduced-fat canola mayonnaise and salt and pepper. Use 2 slices of whole-grain bread. To cut the calories, use only 1 slice of bread and eat open-faced, or stuff into half of a pita.

HOLLY'S CHICKEN SALAD SANDWICH

‖ APPROXIMATELY 455 CALORIES ‖

* 2/3 cup shredded rotisserie chicken
* 1 stalk celery, chopped
* 1 tbsp reduced-fat canola mayonnaise
* salt and pepper, to taste
* 2 slices whole-grain bread

I like this sandwich because it is a great use of leftover rotisserie chicken. I take off the skin and shred the chicken with my hands. Mix ⅔ cup of rotisserie chicken with 1 stalk of chopped celery, 1 tablespoon of reduced-fat canola mayonnaise, and salt and pepper to taste. Use 2 slices of whole-grain bread. To cut the calories, use only one slice of bread and eat open-faced, or stuff into half of a pita.

HOLLY'S TORTILLA WRAP

‖ APPROXIMATELY 180 CALORIES PER WRAP ‖

* 1 low-fat string cheese
* 2 slices turkey bacon
* 1 low-calorie flour tortilla

Tightly roll 1 low-fat string cheese and 2 slices of turkey bacon in a low-calorie flour tortilla. (I use a brand that is 50 calories per tortilla. Check the nutrition label for the calorie information.) Wrap the tortilla in a paper towel and microwave for about 1 to 1½ minutes. This is killer tasty. I usually make two of these for lunch, but you also can have just one with a cup of coffee for a light breakfast.

HOLLY'S COTTAGE CHEESE POTATO

APPROXIMATELY 260 CALORIES

* 1 medium potato
* cooking spray
* salsa, to taste
* 1/2 cup low-fat cottage cheese
* salt and pepper, to taste

Preheat oven to 400°F. Scrub a medium-sized potato, and poke holes in it with a fork. Cook on high in the microwave for about 4 to 5 minutes, or until the potato feels soft when you stick it with a fork. Next, spray the outside of the potato with cooking spray and sprinkle with salt. Bake in the oven for another 5 to 6 minutes, until the skin is crispy. When it's done, cut the potato in half and add ½ cup of low-fat cottage cheese to the middle. Add salt and pepper to taste. You can also top this with salsa. Tasty!

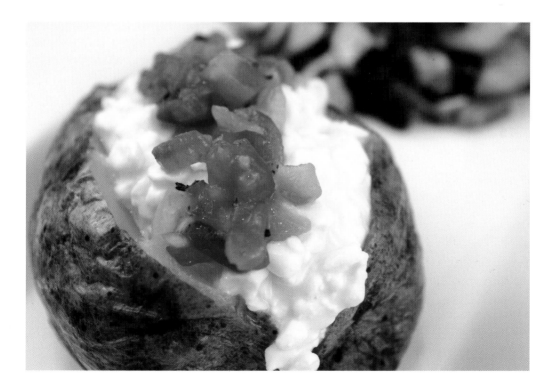

HOLLY'S PITA PIZZA TACO

|| APPROXIMATELY 365 CALORIES ||

* 1 whole-wheat pita
* 1/4 cup spaghetti sauce
* 2 oz low-fat shredded mozzarella

I love this recipe. It's one of my personal favorites. Place a whole-wheat pita on a cooking sheet. Pour ¼ cup of spaghetti sauce on top. Sprinkle 2 ounces of low-fat shredded mozzarella over the sauce. Broil in the oven until the cheese bubbles. Take it out of the oven and let it cool for a minute or two, then fold it in half like a taco. It's easy to eat and tasty! And this is really simple to make into a dinner portion—just add another ounce of low-fat cheese (for 445 total calories). For a variation, you can stuff your Pita Pizza Taco with any leftover Holly's Roasted Veggies (see Side Dishes) also. Yum!

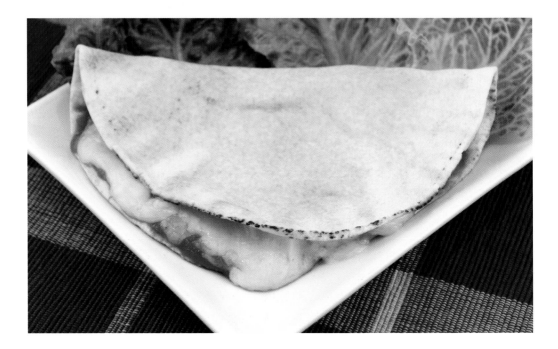

HOLLY'S COTTAGE CHEESE
AND FRUIT SALAD

|| APPROXIMATELY 250 CALORIES ||

* 1 medium pear

* 1 cup low-fat cottage cheese

* 1 pkg sweetener (Splenda)

* cinnamon

Slice 1 medium-sized pear in half and cut out the core. Place both halves, cut side up, on a plate. Scoop 1 cup of low-fat cottage cheese over the pear halves, and top with Splenda and cinnamon. This makes a quick, easy, and very light lunch for days you're planning to go out to dinner and want to have extra calories available, or if you had your pig-out the day before and want to cut calories. You can substitute any low-glycemic fruit, such as cherries, berries, peaches, or plums, for the pears.

HOLLY'S WALDORF SALAD

|| APPROXIMATELY 380 CALORIES ||

* 1 cup low-fat cottage cheese

* 1 small apple, diced

* 6 walnuts, chopped

* 1 oz raisins

* cinnamon

Scoop 1 cup of low-fat cottage cheese into a bowl. Dice 1 small apple. Chop 6 walnuts into small pieces. Measure 1 ounce of raisins (about 50 raisins), and stir the apple, walnuts, and raisins into the cottage cheese. I top this with a little bit of cinnamon. Light, refreshing, and delicious! A great summer lunch.

HOLLY'S BLACKENED CHICKEN SALAD

|| APPROXIMATELY 450 CALORIES ||

* Holly's Rotisserie Chicken (see Dinner Recipes)
* Holly's Salad (see Side Dishes)
* cooking spray
* garlic salt
* pepper
* steak seasoning

I use leftover Holly's Rotisserie Chicken for this recipe after removing the skin and bones. Stir-fry it in a skillet sprayed with cooking spray. Add garlic salt, pepper, and steak seasoning. Continue cooking until the chicken is blackened, then toss into a large Holly's Salad. Yum!

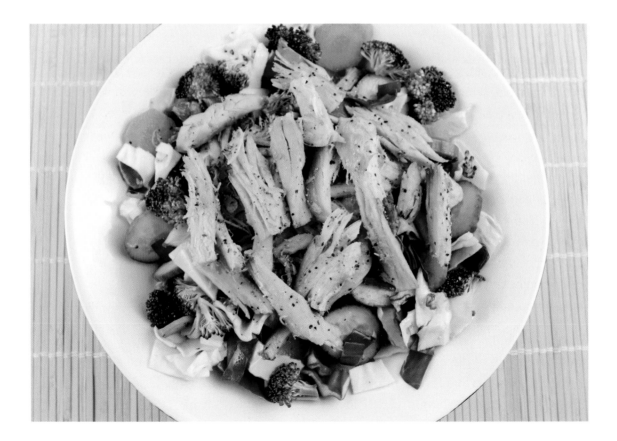

HOLLY'S SHRIMP WITH THAI NOODLES

|| APPROXIMATELY 460 CALORIES ||

* 1 Trader Joe's garlic rice noodle soup bowl
* 10–12 large shrimp
* cooking spray
* garlic salt, to taste
* pepper, to taste

Prepare Trader Joe's garlic rice noodle soup bowl according to instructions. (This is a dry soup to which you add boiling water.) Stir-fry 10 to 12 large shrimp in a skillet sprayed with cooking spray. (I use the frozen shrimp found in the freezer section at Costco.) Flavor the shrimp with garlic salt and pepper to taste. When the soup is done, pour it over the shrimp and simmer together until the soup has evaporated, creating a glaze over the noodles and shrimp. Serve with a large Holly's Salad (see Side Dishes).

Alternative: Stir-fry green cabbage, onion, and garlic, seasoned with salt and pepper to taste, in a skillet sprayed with cooking spray. This cooks down significantly, so go ahead and use at least half a head of cabbage. Serve the shrimp and noodles over the cabbage, either in lieu of the salad or with a salad on the side. If you do not like shrimp, you can substitute precooked grilled chicken strips. I buy packages of these at Costco and Trader Joe's and keep them on hand in the freezer.

HOLLY'S ROTISSERIE CHICKEN WITH SALSA

|| APPROXIMATELY 250 CALORIES FOR A SERVING OF CHICKEN AND SALSA ||

* 1 large precooked rotisserie chicken
* fresh salsa

Buy a large precooked rotisserie chicken from Costco or your local grocery store. Serve with warmed fresh salsa. Be careful to check the calorie count of the salsa, because although the papaya salsas are delicious with this, they are higher in calories. I love the Garden Fresh Gourmet Jack's Special Salsa from Costco (10 calories for 2 tablespoons, so I use as much as I want). Depending on who's eating with us, I serve this with baked potatoes (approximately 130 calories for a small one) or Holly's Rice (see Side Dishes—approximately 120 calories for ½ cup cooked). Serve with Holly's Salad or Holly's Roasted Veggies (see Side Dishes). The kids love it!

HOLLY'S GRILLED SALMON

|| APPROXIMATELY 245 CALORIES FOR A SERVING OF SALMON ||

* 1 marinated salmon fillet
* 1 small sweet potato or yam
* cinnamon
* sweetener (Splenda)

This is a really simple and nutritious meal. I bake 1 marinated salmon fillet. (I use Morey's Marinated Wild Alaskan Salmon that is preseasoned, which I buy at Costco. There are 6 fillets in a box.) The serving is prepackaged, so it is easy to ensure that the calorie count is correct. I serve this with a small sweet potato or small yam (about 150 calories) sprinkled with cinnamon and artificial sweetener (I use Splenda) and Holly's Roasted Veggies (see Side Dishes). This tastes like a restaurant meal. Seriously!

HOLLY'S NACHOS

* 1 can Rosarita 98% fat-free vegetarian refried beans
* 1 cup Holly's Roasted Veggies
* 1 1/2 cups shredded cheddar cheese
* cooking spray
* fresh salsa
* 1 bag tortilla chips

This recipe makes enough for about 3 servings. There are approximately 240 calories in a 1-cup serving of the beans (420 calories in the entire can of beans); the tortilla chips average 10 calories per chip, depending on the brand you use; and make sure to add in the calories for the amount of cheese you eat.

Preheat the oven to 400°F. To prepare, mix 1 can of Rosarita 98% fat-free vegetarian refried beans with 1 cup or more of leftover Holly's Roasted Veggies (see Side Dishes). To save baking time, heat the beans and veggies in a covered bowl in the microwave on high for about 2 minutes. Stir, then spread on the bottom of a glass baking dish sprayed with cooking spray. Place large tortilla chips into the beans. I stick them in at a slant so they stand almost upright. Sprinkle about 1½ cups of shredded cheddar cheese over the top (approximately 685 calories), then bake for about 15–20 minutes. Serve with fresh chunky salsa. I serve this with Holly's Salad (see Side Dishes). This is always a favorite with the guys!

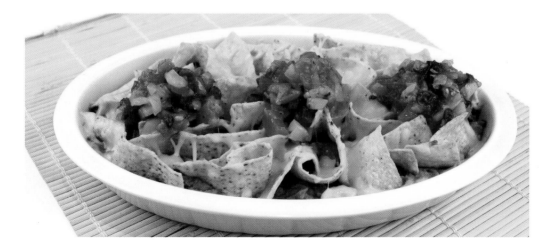

HOLLY'S HIGH-PROTEIN BURGER AND VEGGIES

|| APPROXIMATELY 500 CALORIES FOR THE WHOLE MEAL ||

* 1 preformed burger patty
* steak rub
* Holly's Roasted Veggies
* 1/2 cup low-fat cottage cheese
* ketchup or steak sauce, to taste

I love this dinner. I grill a preformed burger patty (purchased either at Costco or Trader Joe's, they're approximately 280 calories per patty) spiced with our favorite steak rub. Add a healthy serving of Holly's Roasted Veggies (see Side Dishes), and serve with ½ cup of low-fat cottage cheese. Add ketchup or steak sauce to taste.

HOLLY'S SPAGHETTI AND MEATBALLS

|| APPROXIMATELY 550 CALORIES ||

* 2 oz whole-wheat spaghetti
* olive oil
* 1 cup spaghetti sauce
* salt
* 6 frozen meatballs

Boil approximately 2 ounces of whole-wheat spaghetti (about 1 cup when cooked, and approximately 210 calories). I add salt and a drop of olive oil to the water. Microwave 6 small frozen meatballs (I like Trader Joe's frozen Meatless Meatballs; 6 are approximately 140 calories, and they have a lot of protein) and place in a saucepan with spaghetti sauce (1 cup is 160 calories). Heat the sauce with the thawed meatballs, then pour it over the cooked spaghetti. You can substitute regular spaghetti for whole-wheat spaghetti. (If you do this, check the calorie count—it's a little higher.) This is a filling dinner.

HOLLY'S CINNAMON SALMON

APPROXIMATELY 300 CALORIES FOR AN AVERAGE-SIZED SALMON FILLET (50 CALORIES PER OUNCE)

* 6 oz salmon fillet
* cooking spray
* lemon pepper
* cinnamon

You can weigh the fish on a food scale, or even a postage scale—just put some plastic wrap over the scale first.

Preheat the oven to 425°F. Place 1 salmon fillet in a baking dish sprayed with cooking spray. Sprinkle each side of the fillet liberally with lemon pepper, and add a dash of cinnamon. Bake for about 15 minutes or until done. It is delicious!

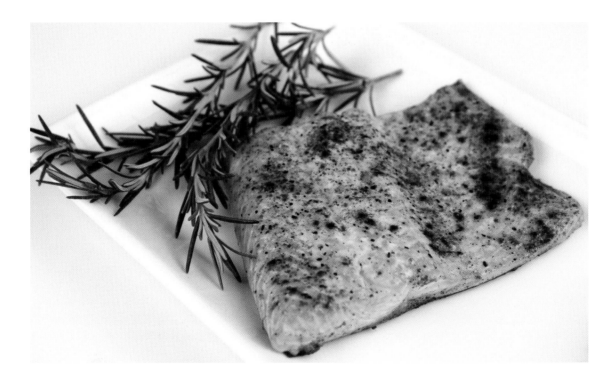

HOLLY'S BAKED PORK CHOPS

|| APPROXIMATELY 300 CALORIES FOR AN AVERAGE-SIZED PORK CHOP ||

* 1 medium pork chop
* cooking spray
* garlic salt, to taste
* pepper, to taste

Preheat the oven to 350°F. Spray the pork chop with cooking spray and season with garlic salt and pepper. Place in a broiling pan sprayed with cooking spray and bake for approximately 20 minutes, then turn it over. Bake for about 15 minutes more, then broil for 5 minutes, just long enough to brown the top. You can serve this with fresh salsa, or it's delicious with Holly's Baked Apples (see Side Dishes) or applesauce, if you have the calories available. I usually serve it with Holly's Microwave Broccoli and Holly's Salad (see Side Dishes).

HOLLY'S CHEESE CANNELLONI

|| APPROXIMATELY 350 CALORIES ||

* 2/3 cup low-fat ricotta
* garlic salt, to taste
* pepper, to taste
* fresh or dried basil (optional)
* 2 crepes
* cooking spray
* Parmesan cheese
* 1/4 cup spaghetti sauce

Preheat the oven to 350°F. In a bowl, mix ⅔ cup of low-fat (not part-skim!) ricotta with garlic salt and pepper. Add fresh or dried basil if you like. Lay 2 crepes out on a cookie sheet lightly sprayed with cooking spray. Spoon half of the ricotta mixture into the middle of each crepe. With each crepe, fold both ends in, then roll it up like a burrito. Bake for about 10 minutes, or until lightly brown. When you take the cannelloni out of the oven, top with ¼ cup of warm spaghetti sauce, and sprinkle Parmesan cheese on top. Yummy!

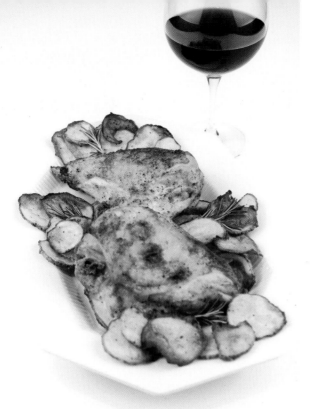

HOLLY'S CURRY CHICKEN BREASTS

|| APPROXIMATELY 300 CALORIES PER AVERAGE-SIZED CHICKEN BREAST ||

* whole chicken breasts
* garlic salt, to taste
* pepper, to taste
* curry powder, to taste
* cooking spray

This is very easy and delicious. Spray a baking dish with cooking spray. Peel away most, but not all, of the skin from fresh, whole chicken breasts. (If you peel away all the skin, the chicken tends to get dry and have less flavor.) Season both sides of the chicken breasts with garlic salt, pepper, and curry. Place the chicken breasts bottom side up in the baking dish. Place under the broiler for about 15 to 20 minutes, until they're cooked and brown on that side. Flip the chicken over and brown the top. It takes about 30 to 40 minutes in all. These taste exotic. I frequently serve them with Holly's Rice or Holly's French Fries (see Side Dishes).

HOLLY'S CHEESY CHICKEN

|| MAKES 2 SERVINGS, APPROXIMATELY 425 CALORIES EACH ||

* 2 boneless, skinless chicken breasts
* 2 slices Swiss or provolone cheese
* 1/2 cup cream of chicken soup or cream of mushroom soup
* 2 tbsp bread crumbs
* splash of wine
* cooking spray

This entrée is quick, easy, and delicious. I serve it to dinner guests. Preheat the oven to 375°F. Spray a baking dish with cooking spray. Place 2 boneless, skinless chicken breasts in the baking dish. Place 1 slice of Swiss or provolone cheese on top of each chicken breast. (Reduced-fat Swiss cheese works well and cuts about 30 calories per slice.) Spoon ¼ cup of either cream of chicken soup or cream of mushroom soup over each breast. Sprinkle 1 level tablespoon of bread crumbs over each chicken breast, then pour a splash of wine over the top of each. I use about an ounce per breast and have used both red and white wine. Bake for approximately 1 hour, or until done. Delectable!

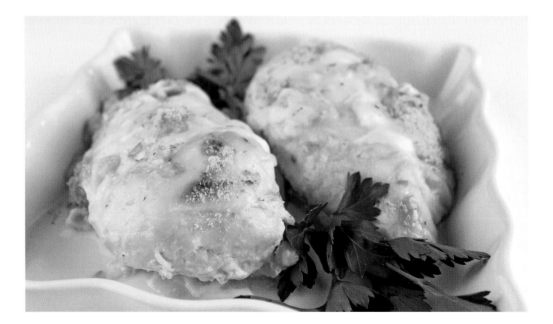

HOLLY'S SALMON PATTIES

|| APPROXIMATELY 220 CALORIES PER PATTY ||

* 6 low-fat, whole-grain crackers
* 2 eggs
* half small onion, diced
* salt and pepper, to taste
* 1 can cooked salmon, 14.75 ounces
* cooking spray

Crumble 6 low-fat whole-grain crackers into a bowl. Add 2 eggs, half of a diced onion, salt and pepper, and blend well. Add 1 can (14.75 ounces) of cooked salmon and mix well. Form into 4 patties. Brown them in a skillet sprayed with cooking spray. If you like salmon, you'll enjoy sandwiches made with any leftover patties.

HOLLY'S STUFFED BAKED POTATO

|| APPROXIMATELY 650 CALORIES FOR A LARGE POTATO ||

* 1 large potato
* cooking spray
* salt, to taste
* 1/2 cup shredded chicken
* 2 slices cheese
* fresh salsa

Preheat the oven to 400°F. Scrub a large potato well, dry it, and poke holes in it with a knife or fork. Cook the potato on high in the microwave for about 5 to 6 minutes, or until it feels soft when you stick it with a fork. Spray the potato with cooking spray and sprinkle it with salt. Transfer it to the oven and bake for another 5 to 6 minutes, until the skin is crispy. While the potato is in the oven, put ½ cup of shredded chicken in the microwave until hot. (I always keep some leftover shredded rotisserie chicken in the freezer to have handy.) When the potato is crispy, cut it in half, place it on a plate, cut sides up, and arrange the chicken over the halves. Place 1 slice of cheese over each half. You can use low-fat cheese if you like. Let the cheese melt, then top with fresh salsa. This is a full meal in itself, and it's killer!

HOLLY'S THOUSAND ISLAND CHICKEN

|| MAKES 2 SERVINGS, APPROXIMATELY 315 CALORIES EACH ||

* 2 boneless, skinless chicken breasts
* 2 tbsp Thousand Island dressing
* 2 tbsp dry onion soup mix
* 2 tbsp brown sugar
* cooking spray

Preheat the oven to 375°F. Spray a baking dish with cooking spray. Place 2 boneless, skinless chicken breasts in the baking dish. Mix 2 tablespoons of Thousand Island dressing with 2 tablespoons of any dry onion soup mix, then add 2 tablespoons of brown sugar and blend well. Spoon the mixture over the chicken. Bake for approximately 1 hour, or until done. Turn the chicken over once during baking, and baste with the sauce occasionally. This is unbelievably tasty and is especially good with Holly's Rice (see Side Dishes).

HOLLY'S FAJITA SALAD

|| MAKES 6 SERVINGS, APPROXIMATELY 400 CALORIES EACH ||

* prepared chicken or steak fajita mix
* 1 large Holly's Salad
* 6 oz shredded cheese
* fresh salsa

This is an easy dish to serve the whole family. Make a large Holly's Salad (see Side Dishes). Prepare chicken or steak fajita filling according to fajita mix package directions. Spoon the salad onto 6 dinner plates, then spoon 1 serving of the fajita meat over each salad. (A serving is ⅙ of the fajita mixture.) Sprinkle 1 ounce or less of shredded cheddar over the top, then top with mounds of fresh salsa. This is not only tasty, but it makes a beautiful presentation. You can also serve the fajita meat mixture in warm corn tortillas with the salad on the side.

HOLLY'S GRILLED STEAK

|| APPROXIMATELY 350 CALORIES PER 6-OUNCE SERVING OF STEAK ||

* 1/2 cup balsamic vinegar
* garlic salt, to taste
* pepper, to taste
* 4 lean steaks (top sirloin or T-bone)

This delicious steak marinade is not only easy, it tenderizes the meat. Mix ½ cup of balsamic vinegar with garlic salt and pepper to taste. Trim the visible fat off 4 of your favorite lean steaks—top sirloin and T-bones are great. Place the steaks in a sealable bag and pour in the marinade. Seal the bag and flip it over a few times to cover the meat. Lay the bagged steaks flat in the refrigerator for 1 hour. Turn them over to marinate for another hour, if possible. Grill until cooked. I'm not a steak lover, but I love this. Fantastic!

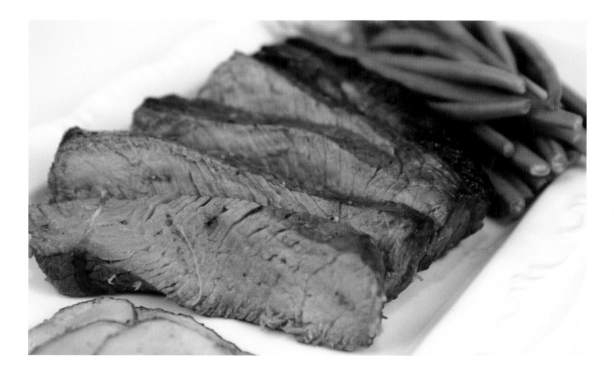

HOLLY'S SIDE DISHES

use cooking spray and just a tiny bit of olive oil (about 1 tablespoon) to coat the skillet when I stir-fry veggies. If the skillet gets too dry, you can always add some water to the skillet as you cook to keep things from sticking without adding calories. And always make sure to wash your veggies well before cooking, even if they come in a package that says "prewashed." It never hurts to be cautious.

HOLLY'S MICROWAVE BROCCOLI

|| APPROXIMATELY 40 CALORIES PER CUP ||

* 3 to 4 cups broccoli, cut into small pieces
* 1 tbsp butter (or butter substitute)
* garlic salt, to taste
* pepper, to taste
* squeeze of fresh lemon juice (optional)

Cut 3 to 4 cups of broccoli into small pieces. Put it in a microwave-safe bowl with a small amount of water on the bottom. Spread a tablespoon of butter (or butter substitute) over the top, and sprinkle with garlic salt and pepper. Cover and cook at full power for approximately 5 or 6 minutes. (Check it frequently, as different microwaves cook at different intensities.) Remove when the broccoli is still a bit crunchy; drain the water, stir, and serve. I particularly like this with lemon squeezed over it.

HOLLY'S SALAD

|| APPROXIMATELY 100 CALORIES PER 2-CUP SERVING* ||

- ✳ romaine lettuce
- ✳ red and green cabbage
- ✳ tomatoes
- ✳ pickling cucumbers
- ✳ broccoli
- ✳ garlic salt and pepper, to taste
- ✳ Italian dressing
- ✳ balsamic vinegar

I use romaine lettuce, red cabbage, green cabbage, tomatoes, pickling cucumbers, and raw broccoli, but you can use any deep green lettuce and low-glycemic vegetables you like—sprouts, bell peppers, onion—but nothing starchy. Sometimes I add a little bit of raw carrot, because even though carrots are higher on the glycemic index, they are full of beta-carotene and antioxidants. First, cut up the veggies and place them in a very large bowl. For dressing, I always start with garlic salt and pepper, then toss with any Italian-type dressing I have on hand. Finally, I add balsamic vinegar. The salad should be lightly coated, but not swimming in dressing. By the way, you can skip the lettuce and the salad still tastes great!

*Calories vary greatly with your dressing choice.

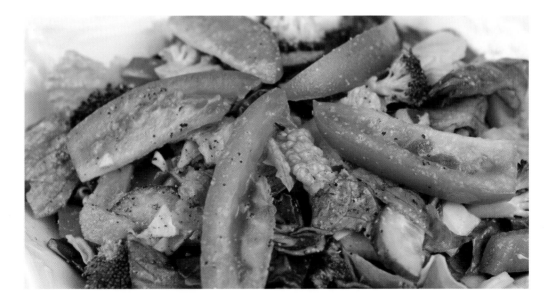

HOLLY'S BROILED TOMATOES

|| APPROXIMATELY 40 CALORIES PER CUP ||

* 2 to 3 tomatoes
* cooking spray
* garlic salt, to taste
* pepper, to taste
* fresh basil (may use dried)
* 1 tsp Parmesan cheese

Thinly slice 2 to 3 tomatoes and place them on a cookie sheet sprayed with cooking spray. Sprinkle with garlic salt, pepper, dried or fresh basil, and approximately 1 teaspoon of Parmesan cheese. Spray the slices with cooking spray and broil for approximately 10 minutes. These taste like pizza!

HOLLY'S MICROWAVE CAULIFLOWER

|| APPROXIMATELY 35 CALORIES PER CUP ||

* 1 head of cauliflower
* 1 tbsp of butter (or butter substitute)
* garlic salt, to taste
* pepper, to taste

This is prepared just like Holly's Microwave Broccoli. Place an entire head of cauliflower in a microwave-safe bowl with a small amount of water on the bottom. Spread about 1 tablespoon of butter (or butter substitute) over the top, and sprinkle with garlic salt and pepper. Cover and cook at full power for approximately 5 or 6 minutes. Remove when still a bit firm; drain the water and serve.

HOLLY'S BAKED APPLES

|| APPROXIMATELY 100 CALORIES PER APPLE ||

* 4 large apples, cored
* cooking spray
* cinnamon
* sweetener (Splenda)

Preheat the oven to 375°F. Core 4 large apples. Spray them inside and out with cooking spray. Sprinkle liberally with cinnamon and Splenda. Bake for 45 minutes to 1 hour, or until soft. I love to serve these with Holly's Baked Pork Chops (see Dinner Recipes). They're so tasty, and they make your house smell wonderful!

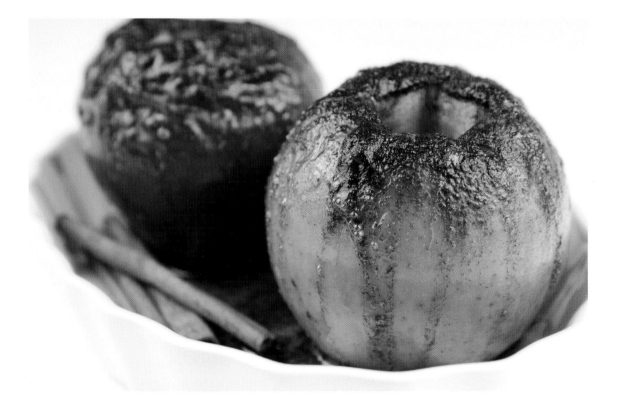

HOLLY'S SPICY GREEN BEANS

|| APPROXIMATELY 45 CALORIES PER CUP ||

* cooking spray
* 1 tbsp sesame oil
* 4 cups frozen green beans
* garlic salt, to taste
* pepper, to taste
* crushed red pepper

Spray a large skillet or wok with cooking spray, and add about 1 tablespoon of sesame oil (you can substitute another oil if you don't have sesame). Heat the oil, then add 4 cups of frozen green beans. I like the French-cut organic frozen green beans you can find at Trader Joe's and sometimes Costco. Add garlic salt, pepper, and crushed red pepper as you stir-fry. I make these beans very spicy, but you can omit the red pepper.

HOLLY'S STIR-FRIED ASPARAGUS

|| APPROXIMATELY 50 CALORIES PER CUP ||

* cooking spray
* 1 tbsp olive oil
* 1 large bunch asparagus
* garlic salt, to taste
* pepper, to taste

Spray a large skillet or wok with cooking spray, and add 1 tablespoon of olive oil. Heat the oil, then add 1 large bunch of fresh asparagus. Add garlic salt and pepper as you stir-fry. Serve when still a bit firm. Although asparagus is not my favorite vegetable, it is filled with vitamins and minerals and rates very low on the glycemic index.

HOLLY'S ROASTED VEGGIES

|| APPROXIMATELY 30 CALORIES PER CUP ||

* 2 or 3 bell peppers
* cooking spray

* 4 to 5 garlic cloves
* 2 cups broccoli florets
* 1 large onion

* 2 zucchinis
* garlic salt and pepper, to taste

This recipe is a big winner in our house. Use any kind of low-glycemic vegetables. I usually use red, orange, and yellow bell peppers, green zucchini, broccoli, onion, and fresh garlic, if I have it on hand. If not, I skip it, and the veggies still taste great. Preheat the oven to 425°F. Cut the vegetables into small pieces. Put them in a large bowl and thoroughly coat them with cooking spray as you stir them around. Add garlic salt and pepper to taste. Place the veggies on a cookie sheet sprayed with cooking spray, and bake for about 20 to 25 minutes, until they are tender and lightly browned. These also taste great left over, so when I make them, I use 2 or 3 bell peppers, 2 zucchinis, 2 cups of broccoli florets, 1 large onion, and 4 or 5 cloves of garlic. This makes two cookie sheets of veggies and gives me plenty of leftovers, either to eat or to use in other recipes like Holly's Veggie Omelet (see Breakfast Recipes) or Holly's Nachos (see Dinner Recipes).

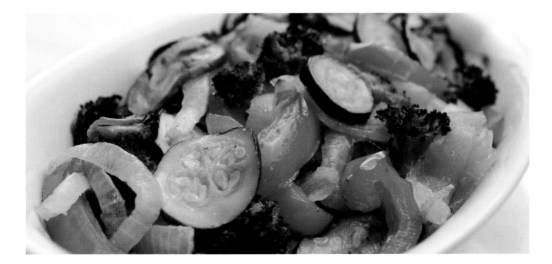

HOLLY'S STIR-FRIED ZUCCHINI

|| APPROXIMATELY 30 CALORIES PER CUP ||

* 4 zucchinis, thinly sliced
* cooking spray
* 1 tbsp olive oil
* garlic salt, to taste
* pepper, to taste

Thinly slice 4 zucchinis. Spray a large skillet or wok with cooking spray, and add about a tablespoon of olive oil. Heat the oil, then add the zucchini. Add garlic salt and pepper as you stir-fry. Serve when still a bit firm. Zucchini, like asparagus, is full of vitamins and minerals and very low on the glycemic index. Plus, zucchini acts as a natural diuretic, helping to rid the body of excess water.

HOLLY'S STIR-FRIED CABBAGE

|| APPROXIMATELY 30 CALORIES PER CUP ||

* 3 to 4 cups of cabbage
* cooking spray
* 1 tbsp olive oil
* garlic salt, to taste
* pepper, to taste

Chop 3 to 4 cups of cabbage. Spray a large skillet or wok with cooking spray, then add about a tablespoon of olive oil. Heat the oil, then add the fresh cabbage. Add garlic salt and pepper as you stir-fry. Use stir-fried cabbage in lieu of a bed of noodles or rice with certain entrées, like a baked boneless, skinless chicken breast or a piece of fish. I frequently do this if I need to cut calories at dinner.